Lords of the Fly

SLEEPING SICKNESS CONTROL IN BRITISH EAST AFRICA, 1900–1960

Kirk Arden Hoppe

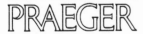

Westport, Connecticut
London

Library of Congress Cataloging-in-Publication Data

Hoppe, Kirk Arden.
    Lords of the fly : sleeping sickness control in British East Africa, 1900–1960 / Kirk Arden Hoppe
        p. cm.
    Includes bibliographical references and index.
    ISBN 0–325–07123–3 (alk. paper)
    1. African trypanosomiasis—Africa, East—History—20th century. 2. Great. Britain—Colonies—Africa—Administration. I. Title.
RA644.T69H67 2003
614.5'33—dc21   2002192187

British Library Cataloguing in Publication Data is available.

Library of Congress Catalog Card Number: 2002192187
ISBN: 0–325–07123–3

First published in 2003

Praeger Publishers, 88 Post Road West, Westport, CT 06881
An imprint of Greenwood Publishing Group, Inc.
www.praeger.com

Printed in the United States of America

The paper used in this book complies with the Permanent Paper Standard issued by the National Information Standards Organization (Z39.48-1984).

10 9 8 7 6 5 4 3 2 1

For TJ

Contents

Figures

Preface and Acknowledgments

I came to the study of colonial sleeping sickness control in East Africa through an interest in fishing on Lake Victoria. I received a Fulbright-Hays in 1992 to study the environmental history of fishing people living around the lake. When I visited archives in Uganda and Tanzania, I found that the early colonial documents mentioning fishing were filed under sleeping sickness. When I spoke to fishers about the colonial period, they spoke of sleeping sickness regulations. People remembered sleeping sickness controls limiting their mobility and economic activities. For many, disease control formed a primary access of their experience with colonial authorities. When I perused colonial maps of the lakeshore, I noted they demarcated sleeping sickness control areas. These maps, oral interviews, and archival documents dramatically illustrated how pervasive controls were in the lives of people living in southern Uganda and northwest Tanganyika. I soon came to recognize the important relationship between colonial disease control and colonial environmental engineering. This book is a result of my discovery of the institutions and ideas comprising this relationship.

The faculty and staff of the Boston University African Studies Center supported my language training in Swahili and my research in East Africa. With Jim McCann, Jean Hay, Sara Berry, Jim Pritchett, and Karl Reynolds on hand, the center was an exciting place for intellectual growth. I would like to thank Jean Allman and Allan Isaacman at the University of Minnesota and Jim Searing, Margaret Strobel, and my colleagues in the Department of History at the University of Illinois at Chicago for their advice and guidance. The Humanities Institute at the University of Illinois at Chicago funded a research trip to Tanzania during the summer of 1999 and a year of thinking and writing in 2000–2001.

In Uganda, Tanzania, and Kenya, the broad-mindedness and largesse of everyone I came in contact with was a blessing and an education in itself. The staff at national and regional archives, at National Fisheries Institutes, and at university libraries in East Africa work hard with little support or remuneration. Academic colleagues in East Africa provided companionship and shared resources. I was graciously hosted in Mwanza by Doug Wilson and Karen Flynn and in Zanzibar by Eric and Donna Gilbert. Craig Harris and David Wiley of the East African Great Lakes Project supplied me with introductions and housing at the Fisheries Institute in Jinja. My sister Dominique and her husband David gave me refuge in Dar es Salaam that refreshed both body and soul.

Friends, family, and colleagues read and reread chapters and provide the inspirations for my intellectual and emotional world. Karen Flynn and Kevin Dunn have been sources of unwavering enthusiasm for my work. Tracey Jean Boisseau was with me in Uganda and Tanzania in 1994 and was involved in every practical and intellectual stage of the project. She is a magnificent mind and spirit and is everything to me.

I owe great debts to the Africans who accompanied me on research trips by canoe, bus, and bicycle, who introduced me into communities, and who translated for me. But I owe my greatest debts to the farming and fishing families in Uganda and Tanzania who had me into their homes and offered me their hospitality and time. It was a great honor for me to meet them and to speak with them. My hosts often asked me why I was asking questions and what my research would mean for them. I told them they would not gain anything in any immediate sense. Though it is my hope that this book in some ways contributes to greater mutuality, I do not imagine that this or the small gifts I could bestow relieves me from the great personal debt to them which I have amassed. I am humbled by their lives, their generosity, and their openness.

CHAPTER 1

Introduction

British sleeping sickness control in colonial Uganda and Tanzania was a powerful mechanism for environmental and social engineering, defining and delineating African landscapes and reordering people's mobility and access to resources. Beginning with the epidemic in Uganda at the turn of the twentieth century that killed perhaps 250,000 people, British disease control officials forcibly depopulated areas infested with tsetse fly and organized African labor to clear vegetation along roads and beaches. Tsetse avoided these cleared spaces, needing the shade and moisture of brush cover. Beginning in the Tanganyika Protectorate after 1920, colonial officials concentrated people in strategically located new villages surrounded by depopulated tsetse areas and had African labor cut and burn large swaths of land as barriers to the spread of tsetse fly between depopulated and settled land.

Lasting until the end of British colonial rule this massive campaign involved tens of thousands of Africans and depopulated thousands of square miles. British scientists and colonial officials saw the spread of tsetse fly, the insect vector of human and animal trypanosomiasis, as a threat to the occupation and potential productivity of African land and to the health of people and livestock. Sleeping sickness officials sought to separate people from tsetse. Regulations abandoned depopulated fly zones to tsetse. Any human presence, except that of colonial scientist-administrators and their African agents, was illegal. In these legally depopulated areas, brush filled in abandoned villages, fields, pastures, and paths and made the land less attractive to future resettlement but very attractive to wildlife and tsetse.

This book is an environmental history of British-colonial sleeping sickness control that examines the social and cultural meanings of depopulations, re-

Figure 1.1
General Area Map

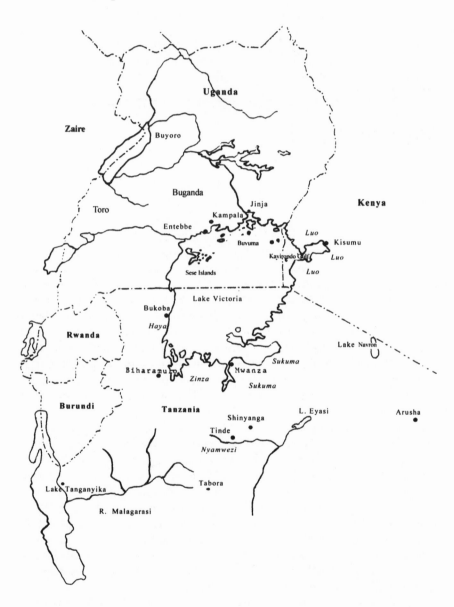

settlement, and brush clearing in East Africa. I make four arguments. My first argument is that the history of colonial sleeping sickness control shows that the emerging Western ideas and institutional powers of public health and colonial development were linked to environmental interventions. In Tanganyika sleeping sickness control was not in response to a particular epidemic, but to fears of rapidly expanding tsetse infestation. Because of the extent of tsetse infestation, officials there did not simply depopulate tsetse areas, but concentrated people in strategically located new villages surrounded by depopulated tsetse areas. By 1934 colonial officials had relocated at least 130,000 people into over 70 sleeping sickness settlements in this area.[1] Within the defensive positions of these theoretically tsetse-free sleeping sickness settlements, colonial agents imagined training local people to live and produce as modern, "rational" farmers and pastoralists. After moral, economic, and medical reeducation, Africans were then to spread back out to reclaim their lands from tsetse in a healthy and orderly manner.

My second argument is that sleeping sickness controls as public health and environmental interventions were central components to the occupation and organization of what the colonial state perceived as economically and politically marginal areas. The British assumed formal colonial control of Uganda in 1900, with an epidemic raging in Busoga. Colonial scientists made the connection between tsetse, protozoan parasites known as *trypanosomes*, and sleeping sickness there in 1903. Medical officials depopulated the Lake Victoria shore and islands, then areas to the north of Buganda, territory often outside direct British and Gandan control, sending people into Buganda. After World War I the epidemic in Uganda abated, and the British continental focus of sleeping sickness research and control shifted to the British protectorate of Tanganyika, newly acquired in 1922. In 1924 colonial officials considered two-thirds of the territory, primarily inland areas remote from colonial political and economic centers, tsetse infested or threatened by infestation. In both colonial Uganda and Tanganyika, colonial officials on sleeping sickness tours were often the first whites to visit and survey communities, and the British implementation of sleeping sickness control was among the first actions of the newly established colonial states in these areas.

My third argument is that the emerging cultural and political authority of natural and medical science informed the logic, organization, and meaning of colonial sleeping sickness control.[2] As colonialism shifted from conquest to occupation, colonial scientists and those employing scientific methods and language had a great deal of leverage and freedom of action at moments when colonial administrations were uncertain about the role and future of colonial rule.[3] European military forces were eliminating primary African resistance, and imperial nations needed new manifestations of power to stabilize occupation and construct morally defensible and economically and administratively viable colonial systems. The new colonial sciences of disease control and development moved into and were structured by this ideological opportunity. Borrowing a term from a scholar of travel literature, Mary Louise Pratt, science served as a form of "anti-conquest." Science was, by definition, not exploitative or oppressive but impartial, absolute, and humanitarian as it claimed to serve the greater human good simply by revealing universal truth through observation. It was "an utterly benign and abstract appropriation of the planet."[4] As an article from the French journal the *Tunisian Review* stated at the turn of the twentieth century, "The doctor is the true conqueror, the peaceful conqueror."[5]

British sleeping sickness control appropriated African environments by envisioning three distinct landscapes: pristine, tsetse-infested, human-free nature; reorganized, tsetse-free human settlement; and man-made, tsetse barriers in between. These were landscapes of science, important in defining and legitimizing colonialism as anti-conquest, where the overarching and transcendent global values of science muted moral questions of forced depopulation, forced labor, and land alienation. Moreover they were important for colonial scientists as areas of relatively unrestricted experimentation, observation, and power. Sleeping sickness control offered scientists from various fields—medical doctors, biologists, entomologists, geologists, botanists, zoologists, as well as colonial disease control policy makers and enforcers—a broad range of opportunities for professional achievement and fame as anti-conquerors. In the fly zones, an early generation of professional natural scientists allied and merged with colonial administrators.

The shift from conquest to occupation, from the authority of the soldier to that of the administrator, rendered the masculinity of the male colonial agent ambiguous. Disease research and control imbued colonial science with a masculinity absent from the image of the scientist as observer of nature and recorder of knowledge. Colonialist stories emphasized the dangers of disease in Africa and scientists' sacrifices for knowledge and the good of Africans. As colonial interventions to improve Africans' physical, economic, psychological, and environmental well-being became grounded in science, they were justified as selfless efforts to protect Africans from themselves and from threatening the environment. The physical danger faced by colonial scientists added an heroic and manly quality to their work.

My final argument is that Africans' actions shaped Western scientific knowledge and the formulation and implementation of colonial policy. Sleeping sickness control is an early example of a high-modernist state project of rationalization and standardization, organizing people and environments, as James Scott argues, according to "state maps of legibility" for efficient surveillance and control.[6] But in practice, colonial sleeping sickness control did not effectively limit the spread of tsetse or control local Africans' activities. Most local people never accepted the logic of the colonial argument for land alienation and restrictions on African movements and activities. They did not abandon depopulated fly areas but reconfigured travel and economic activities.

While colonial sleeping sickness control impacted Africans' relationships to land and resources, local peoples' understandings and responses to policies forced colonial officials to continuously adjust. African responses to forced depopulation and resettlement show the limits of colonial power to order African people and environments. Africans' relationships to sleeping sickness control shifted as people perceived changing threats and opportunities. African farmers, fishers, and local political elite, for example, recognized that resettlement schemes added new variables to a complexity of preexisting relationships and ongoing negotiations over power between family members, between neighbors, between political elite, between political elite and their constituents, as well as between Africans and colonial officials.

Thus Africans' actions shaped systems of Western scientific knowledge as they evolved in colonial contexts. Bridging what might otherwise be viewed as the disparate colonial functions of environmental and health control, sleeping sickness policy by the British was not a straightforward exercise of colonial power. The implementation of sleeping sickness control compelled both Africans and British to negotiate. African elite, farmers, and fishers, and British administrators, field officers, and African employees, all adjusted their actions according to ongoing processes of resistance, cooperation, and compromise. Interactions between colonial officials, their African agents, and other African groups informed African and British understandings about sleeping sickness, sleeping sickness control, and African environments, and transformed Western ideas in practice.[7]

THE ECOLOGY AND HISTORY OF SLEEPING SICKNESS

The perceived epidemiology of sleeping sickness, the ecology of the vectors and reservoirs of the disease, the timing of colonization in East Africa, and the structures of emerging modern Western scientific institutions combined to make sleeping sickness control an important vehicle of colonial intervention. Human trypanosomiasis is known as *sleeping sickness*. While this study focuses on the history of human disease control, livestock trypanosomiasis, known as *nagana*, has an important precolonial and colonial history intertwined with the history of sleeping sickness. Colonial officials understood that nagana drastically limited African pastoralism and therefore potential economic development. Colonial texts often merged concerns about the two diseases under the rubric of sleeping sickness control. Scientists were unclear about differences between the tsetse vectors and trypanosomes for sleeping sickness and nagana and considered both the human and animal diseases as part of the tsetse-borne threat to African productivity and land occupation.[8]

Trypanosomiasis is caused by a blood-borne protozoan infection spread through the bite of the bloodsucking tsetse fly (genus *Glossina*). The parasite trypanosomes enter a fly when it ingests the blood of an infected host, pass through a life stage within the fly, and then infect other hosts when the fly feeds again. Trypanosomes live in the blood and then the central nervous systems of hosts. Currently scientists are unsure of the number of species and subspecies of trypanosomes transmitted by tsetse as well as the number of species of tsetse. Various trypanosomes affect different hosts in different ways and are carried by different tsetse. The primary hosts for trypanosomes are wildlife, livestock, and people. Specific infections may be fatal, or the host may act as a trypanosome reservoir. The trypanosome species *Trypanosoma duttonella vivax* and *Trypanosoma duttonella congolense* produce a disease in livestock similar to that seen in humans but do not harm humans. Domestic animals and wildlife can carry *Trypanosoma brucei rhodesiense*, which is fatal to humans.[9]

The distribution of sleeping sickness is directly linked to the range of the tsetse fly. There are some 20 species of tsetse, 10 of which exist in East Africa.[10] Tsetse expand and contract over 11 million square kilometers of noncontiguous land in Africa.[11] Various tsetse species prefer different, and often overlapping, habitats and food sources. There are lowland rainforest species, forest species, and savanna species of the fly. Water and temperature are important habitat limiting variables for tsetse flies and pupae. Extreme dryness, wetness, heat, and cold are lethal to tsetse. The riverine *Glossina palpalis* species of tsetse, for example, inhabits the shores and rivers of Lake Victoria and needs 40 to 60 percent relative humidity. Temperatures above 40 degrees Celsius and below 16 degrees Celsius are fatal to most species. Vegetation is an important part of tsetse ecology as shade lowers temperatures and holds moisture thereby extending fly habitat in hot, arid regions. Savanna species live along waterways where there is brush cover. Although tsetse species are environmentally sensitive, they move quickly to infest new areas.[12]

The northern range of tsetse is therefore limited by the Sahara Desert to 14 degrees north latitude and by the Somali Desert in southern Somalia to 4 degrees north latitude. Tsetse extend to the edges of the Kalahari 10 to 20 degrees south in the southwest and 20 to 29 degrees south in the southeast. Seasonal low temperatures related to altitude restrict the flies to below 1,800 meters at the equator and to gradually lower altitudes farther north and south.[13]

Not all tsetse carry trypanosomes. In some areas, entire fly populations may not be infected. Scientists do not clearly understand all the factors that influence the distribution of trypanosomes in tsetse. Temperature is one factor. For example, trypanosomes multiply in tsetse only between 25 and 30 degrees Celsius, a narrower temperature range than that tolerated by the fly itself. Normally, however, within a distinct tsetse population, between 10 and 20 percent of flies carry trypanosomes.[14]

Colonial scientists in the early twentieth century identified two types of sleeping sickness, Gambian (or West African) sleeping sickness and Rhodesian (or East African) sleeping sickness, caused by two different species of trypanosomes and transmitted by different species of tsetse. Scientists believed the initial sleeping sickness epidemic in colonial Uganda was caused by tsetse of the species *Glossina palpalis* carrying *Trypanosoma brucei gambiense*, although recent studies call this hypothesis into question.[15] Colonial scientists first identified *T. b. gambiense* in West Africa in 1901 before making the connection between tsetse, trypanosomes, and sleeping sickness in Uganda in 1903.

Then in 1910 in Northern Rhodesia and Nyasaland, British researchers identified a different trypanosome that they named *Trypanosoma brucei rhodesiense* and which was carried by the *morsitans, pallidipes,* and *swynnertoni* species of tsetse. *Rhodesiense* was the primary infective agent among people in Tanganyika beginning in the 1920s. Colonial officials in Uganda in the 1930s and 1940s blamed colonial officials in Tanganyika for not doing enough to control the spread of what they believed was a new kind of sleeping sickness carried by migrant labor from Tanganyika into Uganda.

Early symptoms for both kinds of sleeping sickness in humans include fever, itching, and nausea after the trypanosomes incubate in the blood and lymph. The disease progresses to an advanced stage when the trypanosomes cross the blood-brain barrier and infect the central nervous system. Symptoms then include mental deterioration, seizures, extreme lethargy, sudden and violent mood swings, and sleep disturbance. Death results from complications such as malaria, pneumonia, or dysentery as immune resistance is exhausted, or patients fall into a deep coma and die.[16]

There are important differences between the two types of sleeping sickness involving the historical relationship between people, tsetse, wildlife, environment, and trypanosomes. The difference in habitat between *gambiense*- and *rhodesiense*-carrying tsetse and the difference in the pace of infection influence patterns of transmission.

The trypanosome incubation period for Gambian sleeping sickness is relatively long, taking months to years. Since Gambian sleeping sickness causes chronic infection over a long period, people can function normally for months while carrying the disease, and the disease is often already in an advanced stage when symptoms emerge. The time from infection to death may last several years. *Gambiense*-carrying tsetse live near water. If people regularly access tsetse-infested water sources, over time one infected person can infect a large number of flies who might then infect other people. The transmission of Gambian sleeping sickness is mainly from human-fly-human contact.

In contrast Rhodesian sleeping sickness is more virulent and develops rapidly, usually in a few weeks. The *rhodesiense*-carrying tsetse are savanna species, less dependent on water than the *gambiense*-carrying tsetse. Because the disease develops quickly, infected people are soon incapacitated, resting at home away from wildlife habitat and tsetse. For Rhodesian sleeping sickness, wildlife are the primary reservoir for the disease, and transmission is usually from animals to people. Rhodesian sleeping sickness is more difficult for a person to get and more quickly fatal—death occurs in a few months to within one year.

Without treatment, trypanosomiasis is fatal. Scientists have not yet developed a completely safe and effective drug treatment, although early treatment increases chances of recovery. There is no preventative drug treatment.[17] From 1906 to the present, treatment has consisted of a series of injections of arsenic-based drugs. Different drugs are administered for different types and phases of infection.[18] Although the drugs to treat sleeping sickness—Atoxyl after 1906, Suramine (or Tryparsamide) discovered in 1921, Melarsoprol discovered in 1931, and most recently, eflornithine—have become progressively more effective and less dangerous, treatment has always involved a strict regiment of injections, has never been foolproof, and has serious and often fatal side effects. Tsetse control continues to be the primary method of sleeping sickness control.

Tsetse and trypanosome-carrying wildlife flourish in the savanna brush and forest that fill in abandoned farmlands and pastures. Tsetse withdraw where people clear brush and trees to expand farming and settlement. Sleeping sickness is often endemic among low-density populations of farmers, fishers, pastoralists, and hunters who live near, or regularly move through, tsetse-infested environments. It becomes epidemic at moments of demographic shift when people are either abandoning cultivated areas and pastures or expanding into tsetse-infested brush. In this sense, sleeping sickness is a disease of changing demographic frontiers of human land use in sub-Saharan Africa, and the history of the movement of tsetse fly is linked to the history of the movement of people. Economic and political changes that initiated the movement of people caused the expansions and contractions of tsetse-infested areas in the nineteenth and twentieth centuries. Conversely, the spread and contraction of tsetse influenced the movement of people thus effecting economic and political change.

Historians John Ford (in his formative work *The Role of the Trypanosomiases in African Ecology*), Kelga Kjekshus, and others have documented the history of the spread and contraction of tsetse and sleeping sickness in East Africa. In the late nineteenth century, people abandoned farms and pastures because of warfare, environmental crises, and the spread of other human and animal diseases. Tsetse and trypanosome-carrying wildlife expanded into these areas, and remaining settlers and travelers faced an increased risk of infection. The spread of sleeping sickness in Uganda and Tanzania was a result of the collapse of stable settlement (what John Ford calls "cultivation fronts") that effectively controlled the spread of tsetse.

Economic, political, and environmental changes also resulted in migration into uncultivated areas increasing settler exposure to sleeping sickness until immigrants established stable, tsetse-free fronts. Sleeping sickness expanded in southern Africa as white and African farmers and ranchers aggressively expanded. The Uganda epidemic of 1900 was probably a result of people moving from conflict-, famine-, and disease-ridden areas to the Lake Victoria shore. Increased mobility and population density in an endemic sleeping sickness area sparked an epidemic. Beginning in the 1930s in Tanganyika, Sukuma migration westward into Geita forests and brush resulted first in a sleeping sickness epidemic, then in the contraction of tsetse-infested areas after Sukuma people had cleared enough brush to distance themselves from tsetse.

John Ford's book inspired other historians to reexamine precolonial African disease control and the efficacy of colonial sleeping sickness controls. Ford and others argue that colonial tsetse policies disrupted established African mechanisms for controlling endemic nagana, sleeping sickness, and tsetse, and that forced depopulations probably promoted the spread of tsetse. Africans controlled trypanosomiasis through brush burning, game control, settlement patterns, the careful movement of livestock, and protective ointments for animals.[19] Whether through livestock avoidance or controlled limited exposure, pastoralists in East Africa had sophisticated understandings of tsetse environments and they attempted to control nagana and to limit exposure to tsetse.[20] Richard Waller argues herders in western Narok, Kenya, had methods of expanding into fly-infested bush, first by grazing goats in an area to prepare the way for the final reoccupation by cattle.[21] Gordon Matzke presents evidence that local people in Tanganyika responding to sleeping sickness by dispersing to remote homesteads might have been more effective a mechanism of disease control than the British method of consolidating settlement.[22]

COLONIAL SCIENCE AND TROPICAL DISEASE

The emerging cultural and political authority of science in the West informed the language, logic, organization, methods, and meaning of colonial sleeping sickness control. Western colonialism and Western science are historically connected. Elements of modern science were forged in colonial contexts and applied as a method of imperial power.[23] The methods and ideas of modern science circulated within the colonial world system. In terms of disease control, Western scientists drew upon experiences within Europe and methods used with European populations in formulating disease control policy in Africa and applied experiences and knowledge from Africa in European contexts. Colonial scientists' practices and research methods in Africa were not necessarily different from practice and research in Europe. Western medical interventions were not necessarily more or less brutal and intrusive in Africa than in Europe, nor were Western scientists more or less opportunistic, careerist, or humanitarian in an African versus a European setting. Drug treatment was not necessarily more or less experimental or dangerous for patients on the two continents. But the colonial context of scientific interventions in Africa as opposed to in Europe gave interventions in Africa different cultural and political meanings, and offered scientists broader powers.

Western high imperialism and modern epidemiology emerged side by side. In the 1870s, germ theory replaced the miasma theory of disease that linked disease to the environment and climate. Using the new technologies of the compound microscope and techniques for isolating microbes in laboratory cultures, researchers such as the Pasteurs and Robert Koch successfully isolated particular disease-causing bacilli by 1875.[24] Germ theory and its methods redefined the Western meaning of disease.

The connection between the new science of epidemiology and colonialism is overwhelming. This is obvious in the case of the fields of tropical medicine and tropical disease control, but scientists working in colonial locations also discovered the causes and vectors of diseases common to Europe. Robert Koch isolated the cholera bacillus working in Egypt in the 1870s. Western researchers identified the mode of malaria transmissions in Algeria in 1880 and proved the disease was mosquito-borne in India in the late 1890s. Alexander Yersin and Shibasaboro Kitasato discovered the plague bacillus in Hong Kong in 1894, and Charles Nicolle found the mode of the transmission of typhus while doing research in Tunis in 1909.[25] Western doctors determined how elephantiasis was transmitted in China in 1883 and how yellow fever was transmitted in Panama in 1900.

The institutionalization of tropical medicine was most directly tied to the study of malaria. Medical doctor Patrick Manson published the first comprehensive germ-theory text on tropical medicine, *Tropical Diseases*, in 1898. Manson had shown that elephantiasis was caused by a filarial worm transmitted by mosquitoes. He supported Ronald Ross's research in India in the late 1890s on malaria as a mosquito-borne infection. Manson would become director of the London School of Tropical Medicine, the first medical advisor to the Colonial Office in 1897, and the dominant established voice in early twentieth-century British colonial medicine.[26] Ross, a protégé of Manson, became director of the Liverpool School of Tropical Medicine.

Western imperial states established schools of tropical medicine at the same time they were establishing formal colonial rule in Africa. State and private funds founded the London and Liverpool Schools in 1899, the German Institut fur Schiffs-und-Tropenkrankheiten in Hamburg in 1901, and a school in Brussels in 1906. Tropical medicine was not only a medical specialization but also was structured around natural history, the life cycle of parasites, morphology, and understandings of parasite environments.[27] The Liverpool School's first expeditions were to study malaria in West Africa while the London School focused on malaria in India.[28]

The attention of both schools shifted to sleeping sickness in 1902 with colonial reports of a devastating epidemic in southern Uganda. British politicians and administrators in part saw the epidemic as threatening the political legitimacy of newly established British colonial rule in Uganda (established with the signing of the Uganda Agreement in 1900) in the eyes of African subjects and Western citizens. Colonialists also perceived the epidemic as threatening Ugandan labor needed to translate the imagined wealth of Ugandan environments into colonial exports and British markets in Uganda. In turn politically influential scientists such as Patrick Manson promoted the epidemic in order to expand scientists' power and role in the British empire.[29]

Allan Hoben argues that particular intersections of interests made specific colonial narratives attractive and powerful.[30] The complex epidemiology of sleeping sickness lent control of the disease a broad inclusive allure. Because sleeping sickness control involved environmental issues in depopulated fly areas, economic and social reorganization, and medical testing and treatment, a wide variety of colonial departments involved themselves in the implementation of depopulation and resettlement policy. Sleeping sickness control meetings included representatives from the Tsetse Control Department, Game Department, Health Department, Agricultural Department, Survey Department, Labor Department, and Native Authorities Department. Colonial officials in Tanganyika in the 1940s jokingly referred to sleeping sickness control meetings as "the circus."[31] For officials from various fields and departments, participation in sleeping sickness control linked them to the legitimacy and heroics of colonial science and allowed them to discursively and professionally distance themselves from the violence and contradictory meanings of their actions.[32] Furthermore, the more tsetse spread and the less effective sleeping sickness control was, the more necessary further research and unrestricted scientific interventions became.

SLEEPING SICKNESS CONTROL IN A CONTINENTAL CONTEXT

The Belgians, French, Portuguese, Germans, and British all implemented sleeping sickness research and controls in various African colonies. Before scientists established trypanosome fever and sleeping sickness as the same disease with tsetse fly as a vector of transmission, research on the two maladies was already continentwide. Liverpool School trypanosomiasis expeditions went to Senegambia in 1901 and 1902. The Portuguese state sent a sleeping sickness commission to Principe and Angola in 1901. Reports of the extent and mortality rates of epidemics first in Uganda and then in the Belgian Congo sent waves of concern throughout colonial Africa about the disease as a potential threat to other colonies. Throughout colonial Africa, administrations empowered colonial scientists to meet the ideological and material threats of sleeping sickness. Sleeping sickness control was important in the development of Belgian, French, and British colonial medical services, as well as to the role of science in the ideas and methods of development.

Shared colonial concerns about sleeping sickness led to a degree of scientific internationalism. European sleeping sickness scientists and officials exchanged information and conducted limited tours in each others' colonies. The British promoted an international sleeping sickness bureau at the first International

Sleeping Sickness Conference in London in 1907. The League of Nations sponsored international sleeping sickness conferences and commissions through the 1930s.[33] Nationalism promoted the international sharing of information in the competitive claiming and publishing of scientific "firsts." At the same time, language barriers and national and colonial competition led to degrees of distrust and institutional and administrative separation.

All colonial powers implemented a combination of targeting trypanosomes, tsetse, and people. However, there were distinct differences in approaches to sleeping sickness research and control between the colonial powers. Sleeping sickness control varied also between each European power's colonies and changed within individual colonies over time and according to specific economic and environmental contexts. Sleeping sickness research and controls divided broadly into medical and biological approaches. Each approach involved its own kind of interventions and scientific knowledge, and reflected different colonial relationships to African people and environments. On the one hand, the German scientist Robert Koch emphasized eliminating trypanosomes in people through medical examinations, the isolation of patients, and drug treatment. Medical intervention consisted of research and implementation of treatment, drug cures, and prophylactic injections. The first sleeping sickness drug, Atoxyl, became available in 1906. Colonial doctors identified symptoms and traced how the infection developed and spread through the human body. They carried out patient observation, examinations, segregation, and drug testing in sleeping sickness camps, clinics, and hospitals. Medical controls required mobile medical teams feeling lymph nodes, testing blood, and sending infected patients to quarantined medical facilities.

On the other hand, the British scientist Ronald Ross recommended destroying tsetse, tsetse habitat and food sources, and separating people from flies. A biological approach attacked tsetse-fly infestations through determining and controlling tsetse habitat, behavior, and hosts, including people. Researchers investigated relationships between trypanosome and tsetse types and made connections to human and animal hosts. Biological controls involved environmental interventions to destroy tsetse habitat and to physically separate people from tsetse by moving people away from tsetse or stopping the spread of tsetse into inhabited areas.

In general the British emphasized biological control while the French, Portuguese, Germans, and Belgians pursued medical examinations and drug treatment.[34] Michael Worboys links differences in colonial policies and structures along with differences in scientific advice to three different combinations of sleeping sickness controls he identifies in English-, French-, and German-speaking colonies. According to Worboys, in the first decade of the twentieth century, the British emphasized tsetse control, the Belgians sought to control human movement and space, and the Germans focused on trypanosome control. But while the British and Belgians responded somewhat similarly to epidemics in Uganda and the Belgian Congo with large-scale environmental quarantines to separate infected and noninfected space, once these epidemics died down, the Belgians focused on the medical examinations and treatment while only the British continued to emphasize biological controls.[35]

Worboys mentions that German concerns about labor shortages in German East Africa helped undermine the purely medical approach advocated by Koch. Colonial worries about African productivity and labor supplies generated differences in sleeping sickness control policy between all the colonial powers. In the case of the Congo Free State, the connection between colonial medical institutions and Belgian economic interests was overt. The Liverpool School was founded in 1898 with capital from the Congo Free State consul in Liverpool, Alfred Lewis Jones, whose company held a shipping monopoly between the Congo and Antwerp.[36] The school promoted itself as an investment in increased colonial trade. It advocated minimal intervention and unrestricted commerce as the best way to bring about civilization in Africa.[37]

The Belgian King Leopold II invited a Liverpool sleeping sickness expedition to the Congo Free State in 1903, which declared an epidemic in southern Congo in 1904. The invitation was a public relations maneuver in the face of the growing controversy over colonial atrocities in the Congo Free State and reflected Belgian concerns about disease mortality rates.[38] The sleeping sickness epidemic in the Congo at this time was more geographically extensive than the epidemic in Uganda and resulted in perhaps twice as many deaths.[39] By 1903 in the Congo Free State, colonial profit depended on African access to wild rubber vines and colonial plantations. How Africans organized the environment was less important to rubber companies who were concerned with Africans' abilities to enter forests and extract rubber. Rubber collection necessitated high labor productivity.[40] Sleeping sickness control policies that limited African productivity, disrupted political order, and affected environmental changes conflicted directly with the colonial economic interests in the Congo Free State.

Beginning in 1906, Belgian officials set up cordon sanitaires to monitor and control Africans' movements between infected and noninfected areas and to control African activities that brought them into contact with tsetse.[41] As in Uganda and Tanganyika, there was freedom of movement in noninfected areas, but policed barriers between infected and noninfected areas. Unlike in Uganda and Tanganyika, the Belgian colonial state did not depopulate infected areas. From the onset of controls, however, Belgian administrators argued that compulsory social and economic controls in the Congo were resulting in out-migration and political resistance. As the epidemic ebbed and policy shifted to endemic preventative controls, colonial scientists put the majority of resources into organized medical examinations, segregation of the sick, drug treatment, and mass prophylactic inoculation. Between 1920 and 1923, sleeping sickness medical missions examined 850,000 people and treated 60,000 cases.[42] By 1930, they were examining 3 million people annually.[43] These programs minimized interference in colonial production. Belgian officials experimented on a limited basis with resettlement but they abandoned all resettlement strategies by 1931, claiming the policy was too disruptive politically and economically.[44]

International economic interests also informed Portuguese sleeping sickness control. English merchants put political pressure on the Portuguese government of Principe in response to the sleeping sickness deaths of African cocoa workers. Merchants and plantation owners opposed any restrictions on labor movement and activities. Between 1911 and 1914, Portuguese authorities controlled sleeping sickness on the island through brush clearing, medical examinations, drug treatment, and the destruction of dogs, pigs, and civet cats as potential trypanosome carriers.[45]

The Germans attempted sleeping sickness control in Togo, Cameroon, and German East Africa. In German East Africa, German medical authorities isolated and treated sleeping sickness patients beginning in 1903. The German synthetic drug industry led the West in the development and marketing of antitrypanosome drugs, although the Germans did not implement programs of mass prophylactic injection. Instead, in response to the epidemic in Uganda and the Lake Victoria islands, German authorities were particularly concerned to control movements between the German and British territories.[46] They combined treatment of the sick with mandated examinations of Africans crossing into German territory from British East Africa and Uganda, and bush clearing along these borders and the Lake Victoria littoral.

In the French colonies, as well, sleeping sickness control practices promoted examinations and drug treatment for the sick over environmental controls. The French government sent the first sleeping sickness mission to French Equatorial Africa in 1906 because "the economic future of the Congo is tied to the question of human trypanosomiasis."[47] French nationalists also voiced concern that France not be left behind in colonial medicine. Health authorities issued sleeping sickness regulations in 1909, 1910, and 1911 that mandated health passports for river-steamer travel, bush clearing near settlements, treatment of the sick, and prophylactic treatment for all African employees of concession companies and the state.[48] Albert Schweitzer established a hospital to treat sleeping sickness victims in Gabon in 1913. French medical officials pursued research into drug therapy at the Pasteur Institute station in Brazzaville and organized prophylactic services through a sector system initiated in 1917.[49] Between 1917 and 1919, medical personnel examined 90,000 people in the French Congo. By the 1930s, there were French sleeping sickness teams in Burkina Faso, Ivory Coast, Benin, Senegal, Guinea, Cameroon, and the French Congo.[50]

The French systematically tested and treated Africans throughout French West Africa. French research focused on developing a prophylactic, new drug treatments, and diagnostic procedures.[51] They did not pursue tsetse control in any significant sense. Administrators and concession companies resisted restricting population movements because this disrupted labor supplies, tax collection, and the extraction of coffee and rubber. French administrators in Chad and Equatorial Africa in the 1920s argued that bush clearing and village relocations were unrealistic disease-control policies because Africans fled to remote areas.[52]

In French colonies, as in the Belgian Congo, German East Africa, and Principe, colonial states prioritized natural resource extraction and plantation production. Medical interventions minimized interference with African labor. At the same time, they furthered labor control by locating, counting, examining, and monitoring Africans. While these colonial administrations advocated a combination of trypanosome and tsetse control, they concentrated on eliminating the trypanosome reservoir in Africans through direct medical access.

BRITISH AFRICA

Relative to the rest of colonial Africa, the British were at the forefront of tsetse-control research and implementing policies involving large-scale environmental engineering: fly destruction, fly habitat destruction, game destruction, and human/fly segregation. While the British emphasized tsetse control, the combination of methods control within specific British-controlled territories depended on different colonial economies, environments, and political relationships generating contrasts between British West, Southern, and East Africa. British researchers in Zambia in 1912 identified *trypanosoma rhodesiense*. Beginning that year, sleeping sickness commissions of the Royal Society went to Malawi. British sleeping sickness efforts were made soon after in Northern and Southern Rhodesia and Natal; then they were made beginning in the 1920s in Tanganyika and beginning in the 1930s in Nigeria, Ghana, and the Sudan.

Sleeping sickness control campaigns in Nigeria, Ghana, and the Sudan involved medical examinations, drug treatment, brush clearing, and some limited resettlement. In the 1930s, medical personnel treated 90,000 sleeping sickness cases in Nigeria and administered preventative drug treatments to 300,000.[53] With the exception of the Anchau settlement scheme in Nigeria, tsetse control in West Africa primarily involved clearing and research projects along streams and rivers and unadministered African out-migration from infected areas.[54]

Colonial labor demands created differences in sleeping sickness control methods within British Africa as well. In response to reports from Uganda, in 1908 British officials in Northern Rhodesia instituted drastic resettlement, depopulation, and movement controls for people living to the east of Lake Mweru. By 1910, the state abandoned enforcement in the face of growing demands for mine and railroad labor and in fear that Africans were responding to sleeping sickness controls by migrating to the Belgian Congo.[55] White settler, missionary, and mining interests in southern Africa combined to marginalize sleeping sickness control policies involving depopulations and limits on mobility. Instead, in Malawi, Zambia, Zimbabwe, and Natal beginning at the turn of the century, settler interests in particular promoted game destruction as a method to drive back tsetse and nagana to open new farm and ranch lands. In contrast, the political power of the white-hunter lobby and then nature conservation in Uganda, Kenya, and Tanganyika limited game destruction as sleeping sickness control in eastern Africa.

Within eastern Africa, the history of sleeping sickness control in Kenya stands in contrast to the extensive depopulations and resettlement in Uganda and Tanganyika. The administration and white settlers primarily were interested in the supply and control of African labor to white-settler-owned farms of the central highlands. For the most part, western Kenya was a remote area at the turn of the century, important to the colonial administration only as a transit area to Uganda. Sleeping sickness spread from Uganda to the Kenyan coast and lake islands beginning in 1901. Kenyan medical officials implemented some controls for the islands, for example ordering Mageta Island in Lake Victoria depopulated in 1910 and again in 1921. The Luo and other people living on the shores of Lake Victoria and the Masai in the south resettled by their own accord on higher ground away from tsetse infestation and returned as disease abated. Kenyan officials carried out some tsetse and trypanosome research but usually identified the spread or contraction of sleeping sickness and nagana after local people had already adjusted to the disease. Clearing experiments and projects were confined to riverbeds.

As the Luo became an important migrant labor force for Nairobi and colonial plantations in the 1920s, Kenyan officials implemented medical examinations and drug treatment for labor. Medical officers examined all labor passing through Kisumu and other western recruitment centers for sleeping sickness. Between 1922 and 1926, medical officers cleared 73,500 workers recruited by labor agents.[56] But the Kenyan state did not restrict movement or concentrate populations as it did in Uganda and Tanzania, and Kenya was never important to scientific sleeping sickness research efforts.[57]

RESETTLEMENT, PUBLIC HEALTH, AND SOCIAL CONTROL

British East African sleeping sickness control was unique with its emphasis on large-scale planned human resettlements. Plans for these settlements incorporated emerging ideas about public health. By the 1930s, colonial officials envisioned carefully designed sleeping sickness settlements as sites for the comprehensive modernization of African economies and activities to promote health. Disease prevention in the case of sleeping sickness necessitated controlling Africans' movement to limit exposure to tsetse and controlling Africans' economic activities to create tsetse-free environments. Sleeping sickness officials made a fundamental public health argument that Africans' economic behaviors influenced how vulnerable they were to disease and that the comprehensive restructuring of production systems and work habits was essential to disease control.

While ideas of public health were new to resettlement projects, from the Romans to the Aztec there is a long history of empires using forced resettlement as a mechanism of social and environmental control. In the twentieth century such projects often employed the metaphor of an infectious threat necessitating defensive resettlement. In the 1950s the British colonial state explained moving civilians to barricaded villages in Kenya in part in terms of keeping them safe from the psychological disorder of Mau Mau.[58] In the 1960s the U.S. government promoted the policies of strategic hamlets in South Vietnam as protecting civilians from the spread of communism.[59] In the Soviet Union and postcolonial Cambodia, Tanzania, Ethiopia, and Mozambique, states justified forced resettlement campaigns as promoting national identity and progress in the face of localism, disunity, backward political thinking, and nonrational economic behavior. Such schemes allowed for quicker and more efficient state surveillance, taxation, and control of production and personal behavior.[60] Certainly East Africans' responses to resettlement included fears that living in the new villages would bring them under the eye and thumb of the colonial state.

Colonial states in Africa attempted a wide variety, in terms of scale, organization. and purpose, of resettlement schemes. Most were not compulsory and involved state visions of agricultural modernization, demographic adjustments to overpopulation, dam building, and land alienation by white farmers, miners, naturalists, and engineers.[61] The majority of these projects were failures in terms of improving economic and social conditions for their residents. Sleeping sickness resettlement was the most extensive of these schemes in terms of longevity, geography, and the number of settlers involved. It provided a model and testing ground for a broad spectrum of ideas about economic and environmental restructuring applied to development projects throughout the globe. Data, reports, and analysis by sleeping sickness officials circulated amongst a globally mobile community of Western scientists and policy makers.

The success of settlement schemes depended on restructuring Africans' actions. In the conception, implementation, and analysis of settlement schemes, colonialists developed and tested technologies of environmental surveying, human surveillance, and project evaluation. Tsetse surveys mapped the exact location, occupation, and movement of local people and the location of resources. Officials used geological surveys, maps of vegetation types and water sources, and soil studies to dictate where Africans could and could not live.

ENVIRONMENT AND MEANING

The meaning of colonial sleeping sickness control is reflected in the production, consumption, and interaction of three separate and interconnected bodies of texts: colonialist texts, African texts, and texts that reveal the interactions between local people and colonial agents. Colonialist texts about tsetse and sleeping sickness reflect discussions among and between colonial scientists, colonial officers, politicians, and within popular culture in Britain and the West. Sleeping sickness and tsetse had an important and powerful meaning for colonialism. Because of the environmental nature of British sleeping sickness control, it involved imagining African environments and Africans' place in those environments.

Development theorist Emory Roe argues the importance of development master narratives in stabilizing and underwriting the assumptions necessary for (in this case colonial) decision making.[62] The story framing British colonial sleeping sickness control policy was that disease-carrying tsetse fly were rendering Africa uninhabitable and unproductive because local people were not effectively occupying land.[63] British understandings of African environments and of African relationships to the environment in this story were important factors in the formulation and enforcement of colonial sleeping sickness control policies as environmental intervention. The British based sleeping sickness control policy on their perception of tsetse-infested areas as wilderness and on understandings of Africans' relationships to these environments as impermanent and insubstantial. British visions of East African environments connected political and economic order with health, and connected mobility, political, economic, and environmental disorder with disease. This story colored British views of the bodies and behavior of Africans and of African lands and informed British perceptions of Africans' responsibilities and rights. In East Africa, the same story played itself out in different ways in Uganda and Tanganyika, reflecting a dramatic contrast in Western discussions between the productivity, wealth, and order of Uganda and the poverty and desolation of northwest Tanganyika.

The British narrative of Africans' relationship to nature was generated, reinforced, and questioned by intersections between scientific, political, and popular knowledge. Each genre of knowledge drew from the others for cultural power and prestige. For example, the actions of colonial officers in the field did not occur in cultural isolation from popular Western travelogues about Africa published in London and New York. The two kinds of stories responded to and built upon one another.

Africans negotiated within the colonial visions of the British officials, often carefully situating themselves and their relationships to African lands in response to opportunities that colonial environmental interventions presented. Just as colonialists understood sleeping sickness control policies in a context of economic, political, professional, and ideological interests, so too did Africans consider colonial controls in the context of their own economic, political, and ideological interests. African individuals and groups evaluated a complexity of interconnected and sometimes contradictory variables in their negotiations over sleeping sickness control. When African elite made strategic decisions about whether or how much to support colonial policies, they considered their political relationships to their own constituencies. African farmers and fishers strategically maneuvered through sleeping sickness control to redefine power relations with local African elite, to abandon one chief for another, or to assert an independent political identity by settling illegally in legally depopulated sleeping sickness areas. On the level of the family homestead, moments of forced relocations were opportunities for some family members to establish independent homesteads in new areas, to take up new professions, or to join the migrant wage-labor force.

A third textual focus involves the interaction between local people and colonial agents. This is in part the history of African colonial employees whom historian Nancy Hunt calls "cultural middles."[64] But colonial field officers and local elite were also in the middle, if in between different things. Colonial field officers read general policy and then interpreted it in specific contexts with particular resources and relationships with local people. Officials did this depending on their changing relationships to colonial administration on the one hand, and African power on the other. And local elite acted as middles between their constituents and colonial agents. The British negotiated with Africans as organizers, enforcers, laborers, medical examiners, patients, and settlers over the implementation of sleeping sickness control. Conversations and experiences in the middle included local people and control officers talking together at village meetings, British men touching Africans during medical examinations and treatment, Africans and colonialists observing one another during organized brush clearing, Africans petitioning colonial officials in protest, and officials punishing African resisters.

Evidence from colonialist and African texts are fractured and sometimes self-contradictory. Interest groups combined and competed for resources and power within and across ethnicity, status, and gender. This colonial history is an examination of the multiple meanings within colonial interactions. Africans and Britons had divergent understandings of sleeping sickness control schemes, nature, and colonial order in East Africa from 1900 when the colonial business of sleeping sickness began through the end of the colonial period. The relationship between African responses (or nonresponses), shifting colonial perceptions of Africans and African environments, as well as the practical limits of colonial power to order African people and environments determined the impact and meaning of sleeping sickness control interventions in restructuring African landscapes and lives.

OVERVIEW

Viewed in combination, British scientific and popular literature together with archival colonial sources and African oral sources illuminate the multiple meanings of colonial sleeping sickness control. National and district archives in Uganda and Tanzania contain colonial reports, letters, and logs showing how colonial officers understood African relationships to environment, how Africans affected the colonial application of sleeping sickness controls, and colonial officers' understandings and reactions to African actions. These archives also include African letters and petitions to colonial officials.

I conducted oral interviews in 1993, 1994, and 1999 in former sleeping sickness areas in the Lake Victoria basin of Uganda and Tanzania. My archival and oral evidence from Uganda focuses on the Lake Victoria littoral and islands in the northern lake. In late 1993, I hired local translators to help me interview people on Sigulu, Bavuma, and Mpuga Islands, and in south Busoga near the lakeshore between Jinja and the Ugandan border with Kenya. All these locations were epidemic areas at the turn of the century and were part of depopulated colonial sleeping sickness areas.

My Tanzanian oral interviews and archival sources focus on the corridor in northwest Tanzania between Lake Victoria and Lake Tanganyika, including Mwanza, Shinyanga, and Kigoma Districts, which was also a primary focus for British colonial sleeping sickness control. In Tanzania in 1994 and 1999, again through local translators, I gathered information from people living on Ukerewe Island and living in former sleeping sickness settlements in Geita and Biharamulo Districts near the southern shore of the lake: Katoro, Biharamulo, Bwanga, and Nyankumbu. Occupied by Ha, Zinza, Sumbwa, and Sukuma groups, these areas were remote from colonial political and economic centers and contained many of the planned sleeping sickness resettlements and brush-clearing schemes in Tanganyika.[65] Close to 80 percent of the total tsetse territory reclaimed in the Tanganyika Territory by depopulation and brush clearing was in the Lake Victoria Basin—in Lake, Central, and Western Provinces.[66]

In both Uganda and Tanzania, translators helped me conduct individual and group interviews principally with elderly men and women. I communicated with my translators in English and Swahili while they spoke with local people in the variety of languages: Swahili, Sukuma, Luo, Luya, Ha, Baganda, Basoga, and others. Local people's memories of the 1920s and 1930s were often childhood memories of depopulations and resettlement or secondhand stories they had heard from their parents and older family members.

Luise White's distinction between "contextualizing testimony rather than 'letting Africans speak for themselves,' " is compelling as I consider African oral sources and colonial written sources in light on one another.[67] As Luise White notes, "To use both sets of sources to produce two separate narratives would ignore the extent to which the subject of the narratives was the same—

that is, both describe the encounter between medical workers and Africans. Moreover, this evidence cannot be separated into discrete units; the oral invades the written too much for that. Instead, I want to suggest that they refract, that they provide ways to read each other."[68] This process of refraction involves the variety of strategic responses by Africans and colonialists that I discuss in the previous section. While African and British sources on sleeping sickness control often contrast with each another strikingly, they do not reduce to two distinct opposing positions, one the unified oppressed and the other the unified oppressor, or one legitimate local knowledge and the other illegitimate knowledge imposed from without. Rather they represent ongoing conversations between local, regional, and global forces.

Furthermore, local people's stories, as well as colonialists' memoirs, travelogues, reports, and letters were forged in the context of the entirety of their life experiences and particular socioeconomic positions, and for the people I interviewed through their understandings of my position and intentions. In Katoro, Tanzania, Salvatory Kalema, an elderly man who lived on a poorer homestead off the main road, told me that before being resettled to Katoro, British officers had promised him and his neighbors that the colonial government would make material investments in the new community. Salvatory bitterly reported that the British had delivered nothing. His neighbor of similar age, Rutekelayo Ifunza, owned a small café and boarding house on the main road. Rutekelayo emphasized that resettlement had concentrated people along the road and therefore had promoted economic opportunity.[69] The men's contrasting economic situations in the present might have informed their perspectives on the past.

In both Uganda and Tanzania, people connected my interest in the history of sleeping sickness control to issues of contemporary land tenure and state power. As sleeping sickness control involved and continues to involve state alienation and reallocation of land, current issues and tensions over land tenure and state authority impacted on discussions about the past. At the former site of the sleeping sickness camp at Busu in south Busoga, some local people reacted to my visit, my questions, and my requests for interviews with consternation and anger. They refused to speak to me or to show me the location of the former camp and accompanied me en masse to the home of James Mwanga, a local political leader. James Mwanga explained to me that the group feared my questions might lead to the state reclaiming formally depopulated state-controlled sleeping sickness land where they now lived.[70] At that time the Ugandan state was evicting people from newly designated forest reserves.

Most of the people I interviewed were men. Usually I took directions and advice from local leaders as to with whom I should speak. Community leaders were almost entirely male and these men directed me to other men. Even when working with female translators, local men asserted themselves to speak with me first. I often felt comfortable asking women for interviews only after

I had spoken with the men in the household who initially approached me. In short Africans' responses to my whiteness and my maleness and my own responses to Africans' gender informed the interviewing process.

In the colonial period, sleeping sickness officials were male and employed only African men as fly boys, fly guards, and medical personnel. African women experienced resettlement, medical examinations, and the absence of conscripted male brush-clearing labor, but the process of resettlement prioritized African patriarchal power. Officials negotiated with local male leaders over resettlement, distributed new farms, tools, and seed to African men, and gave men official control over the markets, courts, policing, churches, schools, clinics, and extension programs in planned settlements.

This history of British sleeping sickness control in East Africa follows chronologically and geographically research, policy making, and control actions from their beginnings through the end of colonial rule in Tanzania and Uganda. The chapters move from the Ugandan epidemic at the turn of the century to Tanganyika beginning in the 1920s, then to the implementation in Uganda and Tanganyika of policies developed at the tsetse research headquarters in Shinyanga, Tanganyika. The Ugandan epidemic paralleled the beginning of formal British colonial control in Uganda in 1900. As this epidemic died out, the center of British research and control shifted to the Tanganyika Protectorate in the early 1920s, again paralleling the beginning of formal British colonial rule there.

Chapter 2 examines the importance of the sleeping sickness epidemic in Uganda to the rise of colonial science as a profession and as a method and ideology of occupation. Beginning in Uganda in 1903, tsetse control and sleeping sickness were important symbols for the legitimacy of colonial intervention and for Western cultural understandings of Africa. I connect British sleeping sickness control to political meanings of the perceived fertility and environmental and political order in the Buganda Kingdom in contrast to the perceived disorder in neighboring areas. African and British understandings of local landscapes, local political and production systems, and British colonial agendas and relationships to African states shaped the colonial meaning of sleeping sickness and the forms sleeping sickness control took. The Ganda state exercised a great deal of power in where and how colonial sleeping sickness control occurred, and the Ganda-British alliance promoted sleeping sickness and Ganda imperial aspirations.

Chapter 3 explores the environmental and geopolitical effects of sleeping sickness control in Uganda through 1920 when the British declared the threat of the epidemic over in most areas. British disease control officials ordered large parts of Uganda depopulated between 1906 and 1914 to separate people from tsetse. Sleeping sickness policies strengthened Ganda regional power by depopulating politically marginal and resistant areas around the center of Buganda. Sleeping sickness control relied on Ganda police, officials, and trained employees to conduct research and implement policy in Buvuma, Busoga, and

Bunyoro, areas whose populations were historically hostile to Ganda author-ity. Controls restructured local peoples' relationships to environments and resources.

After 1922 former German East Africa became the British protectorate of Tanganyika and the primary center of British sleeping sickness research and control in Africa. The shift to Tanganyika included an important reorientation from epidemic control to preventative tsetse-fly control. In contrast to how colonialists perceived Uganda, colonialist images of northwest Tanganyika were of environmental and political desolation and disorder. In chapter 4 I connect these images to the career of Charles Swynnerton, the first game department director and tsetse control director in Tanzania. The emerging ideas of nature conservation influenced Swynnerton's approach to sleeping sickness control and the research agenda at the 800-square-mile tsetse-control research station at Shinyanga. His research methods and control policies com-bining depopulation, brush clearing, and planned resettlement became models for the rest of British Africa.

In 1935 the tsetse committee in London supported Swynnerton's argument for planned sleeping sickness settlements. Chapter 5 presents the local me-chanics of the implementation of depopulations and resettlements in Tan-ganyika after 1935, when officials carefully designed settlements to control Africans movements, economic activities, and social organization. There was a general British colonial shift in the mid-1930s to more comprehensive co-lonial development initiatives involving comprehensive social and environ-mental control. A second epidemic in southern Busoga in 1940 and the continued spread of tsetse there brought renewed control efforts to Uganda as well.

Colonialists were uncomfortable with land alienation, forced resettlement, and brush clearing as part of the colonial civilizing mission; sleeping sickness control actions appeared neither civilized nor civilizing. Chapter 6 follows colonial discussions that sought to mitigate moral contradictions about forced labor for brush clearing and to justify depopulation and land alienation. Co-lonialists argued that local people didn't mind relocating, that Africans were used to coercion and did not value free labor as Westerners did, and that Africans were to blame, in part, for sleeping sickness and the spread of tsetse. Faced with ongoing African resistance and the continuing spread of tsetse, colonialists in the 1930s began to emphasize that as opposed to being a threat to African livelihood and health, tsetse were more important in protecting African landscapes from African misuse. Connections between nature con-servation and tsetse control are reflected in the overlapping geographies of depopulated fly zones and conservation areas.

The implementation of sleeping sickness control policy was not consistent or, from the perspective of the colonial state, successful. Controls did not effectively limit the spread of tsetse or prescribe local Africans' activities. Lo-cal people resisted, negotiated with, and manipulated sleeping sickness control officials in the context of local power relations. Chapters 3–6 examine African experiences of sleeping sickness control and follow British adjustments, in ideology and action, to African responses. African responses to forced depopulation, resettlement, and forced clearing labor show the limits of colonial power to order African people and environments. Africans' relationships to sleeping sickness control shifted moment to moment as people perceived changing threats and opportunities. African farmers, fishers, and local political elite, for example, recognized that resettlement schemes added new variables to a complexity of preexisting relationships and ongoing negotiations between family members, between neighbors, between political elite, between political elite and their constituents, as well as between Africans and colonial officials.

NOTES

1. Kjekshus, 170–172.
2. Jean Comaroff, "The Diseased Heart of Africa: Medicine, Colonialism, and the Black Body," in Lindenbaum and Lock, 306; Vaughan; Lyons, *The Colonial Disease*.
3. Grove, *Green Imperialism*, 7; also see Vaughan, 21, and Richard H. Grove, "Early Themes," in Anderson and Grove, 22.
4. Pratt, 38–39.
5. Quoted in Gallagher, 11.
6. Scott, *Seeing Like a State*, 3.
7. White, "Victims Dull," 1379–1402.
8. Jahnke: Mulligan.
9. Hide et al., 95–111.
10. Knight, 23–44; Glover, 581–614.
11. Jordan, 15.
12. C. G. N. Mascie-Taylor, "Introduction," in Mascie-Taylor, 9–10; Knight, 31–32.
13. Jordan, 15–23.
14. Ibid., 23.
15. Koerner, de Raadt, and Maudlin, 303–306.
16. Knight, 28.
17. Glover, 609.
18. World Health Organization, *Human African Trypanosomiasis* (2002).
19. Kjekshus; Singida, 183–187.
20. Waller, 81–101; Giblin, 59–80; Matzke, "Settlement and Sleeping Sickness Control," 209–214; Matzke, "Reassessment," 531–537.
21. Waller, 81–101.
22. Matzke, "Reassessment."
23. Lindenbaum and Lock, 306; Vaughan; Summers, 787–807; Lyons; Frantz Fanon, "Medicine and Colonialism," in J. Ehrenreich, ed., *The Cultural Crisis of Modern Medicine* (New York, 1978); White, "Tsetse Visions," 219–245; Arnold, *Imperial Medicine*; Gallagher; Marks.
24. Gallagher, 12–13; M. Worboys, "Manson, Ross and Colonial Medical Policy: Tropical Medicine in Liverpool and London, 1899–1914," in Roy Macleod and Milton

Lewis, eds., *Disease, Medicine and Empire* (London, 1988), 22–23; Oliver Ransford, *Bid the Sickness Cease* (London, 1983), 78–81.

25. Gallagher, 6–7.

26. Worboys, "Colonial Medical Policy," 26–27; Manson-Bahr.

27. Worboys, "Colonial Medical Policy," 21–22.

28. Lyons, 68–69.

29. Summers, 787–790; Haynes.

30. Allan Hoben, "The Cultural Construction of Environmental Policy," in Melissa Leach and Robin Mearns, eds., *The Lie of the Land* (Oxford, 1996), 186–208.

31. Tanzania National Archive (TNA), Dar es Salaam, Tanzania, T5/1/1, 1 August, 1950.

32. Haynes, 468, 473.

33. Worboys, "Comparative History," 98; Helen Tilley, "Africa as a 'Living Laboratory,'" (unpublished D-Phil, Oxford University, 2001).

34. Lyons, 102–103.

35. Worboys, "Comparative History."

36. Lyons, 69–70.

37. Worboys, "Comparative History," 26–27.

38. Lyons, 73–75.

39. A. J. Duggan, "An Historical Perspective," in Mulligan, xlix.

40. Headrick, 312.

41. Lyons, 103.

42. Duggan, l.

43. Lyons, 103.

44. Ibid., 215–219.

45. John McKelvey, *Man Against Tsetse: Struggle for Africa* (Ithaca, 1973), 114–120.

46. Kjekshus, 168; Stendel, 434–447.

47. Martin Leboeuf Roubaud quoted in Headrick, 77.

48. Headrick, 89–90.

49. Ibid., 346.

50. Duggan, lix.

51. Ibid., 312–313.

52. Raphael Antonetti quoted in Headrick, 366.

53. Duggan, lix.

54. Duggan, lii; T. A. M. Nash, *Tsetse Flies in British West Africa* (Colonial Office, 1948); T. H. Davey, *Trypanosomiasis in British West Africa* (Colonial Office, 1948).

55. Musambachime, 160.

56. Kenya Annual Medical Report, 1926, Zanzibar Archives (ZA), Zanzibar, 41.

57. Kenya Annual Medical Report, 1920, 1925, ZA; Marc Dawson, "Socioeconomic Change and Disease: Smallpox in Colonial Kenya, 1880–1920," in John Janzen and Steven Feierman, eds., *The Social Basis of Health and Healing in Africa* (Berkeley, 1992), 98; Marc Dawson, "Health, Nutrition, and Population in Central Kenya, 1890–1945," in Dennis Cardell and Joel Gregory, eds., *African Population and Capitalism* (Boulder, 1987), 201–217; Lewis, "Part I," 183–189; Lewis, "Part II," 9–14; Lewis, "Part III," 74–79; D. H. H. Robertson, "Yala River."

58. Susan Carruthers, *Winning Hearts and Minds: British Governments, the Media and Colonial Counter-Insurgency, 1944–1960* (London, 1995).

59. Milton Osborne, *Strategic Hamlets in South Vietnam: A Survey and a Comparison* (1968, Ithaca).

60. Scott, 3.

61. Chambers.

62. Emory M. Roe, "Development Narratives, Or Making the Best of Blueprint Development," *World Development* 19, 4(1991), 120.

63. Ford, *African Ecology*, 6.

64. Hunt.

65. Kjekshus, 170–172.

66. Swynnerton, *The Tsetse Flies of East Africa;* Ford, *African Ecology*, 202; S. Napier Bax, "A Practical Policy for Tsetse Reclamation and Field Experiment," *East Africa Agricultural Journal*, 9(1944); Tsetse Research and Reclamation Department Reports, 1949–1960, ZA.

67. White, "Victims Dull," 1381–1382; also see L. White, *The Comforts of Home: Prostitution in Colonial Nairobi* (Chicago, 1990), 21–28.

68. White, "Victims Dull," 1383.

69. Interview with Salvatory Kalema, Katoro Village, Geita, Tanzania, September 15, 1994; Interview with Rutekelayo Ifunza, Katoro Village, Geita, Tanzania, September 15, 1994.

70. Interview with James Mwanga, Busu, Uganda, January 9, 1994.

CHAPTER 2

The Scramble for Sleeping Sickness: Imperial Interests and the Rise of Colonial Science

Concurrent with the British colonization of Uganda, people living near the northern shore of Lake Victoria in the region of Busoga were dying in increasing numbers from a disease epidemic. By 1905, the colonial state estimated the number of deaths in southern Uganda at over 200,000.[1] The timing, perceived drama, location, and epidemiology of the sleeping sickness epidemic in Busoga combined to give colonial African sleeping sickness control an important role in influencing public health, medicine, natural science, colonial politics, and environmental interventions in British East Africa and throughout colonial Africa.

The British politics of colonialism converged on this epidemic, making sleeping sickness a top priority and focal point for scientific research and colonial intervention. Half-submerged goals of these politics included the justification of colonial expansion in Africa, the establishment of colonial power in Uganda specifically, and the increased professionalization and augmentation of Western science. The Royal Society of Medicine in England sent teams of European scientists to Uganda beginning in 1902 to investigate the epidemic. In 1903 Royal Society researchers connected the epidemic to the protozoal infection of trypanosomes spread through the bite of the tsetse fly. The disease became a symbol in Western understandings of Africa and the civilizing mission and a vehicle for the emerging political and cultural power of colonial science.

Colonial sleeping sickness controls also reflected African understandings of environment and disease, and varied according to African responses to colonial interventions. This chapter explores the African and European ideas and institutions that informed British responses to the sleeping sickness epidemic in Busoga and influenced British and African understandings of subsequent British sleeping sickness research and control in Uganda. The geographies of Ganda imperialism and of British sleeping sickness control in Uganda at the turn of the century overlap. There are environmental and political reasons for this overlap. Ganda and then joint British-Ganda actions along with a confluence of environmental events affected where tsetse and sleeping sickness occurred. The organization and political interests of the Ganda state and of people living in areas impacted by sleeping sickness controls influenced British presuppositions about the relationships between political order, disease, and environment and influenced how local people responded to colonial disease control interventions. Africans affected how and where sleeping sickness control occurred as well.

For British colonialism, the imagined economic potential of the new colony lent importance to sleeping sickness control. The Ganda state impressed Westerners with its control of productive people and of lush environments. Nineteenth-century colonial texts characterized the lands north of Lake Victoria as quintessential tropical exuberance: relatively high, evenly distributed annual rainfall, fertile soils, and hardwood forests. They presented diverse and abundant peasant production well-managed by the kingdom of Buganda.

The value of Uganda in British colonial politics and imperial culture made the sleeping sickness epidemic both a challenge and an opportunity for emergent professional scientists and for the new ideas of constructive imperialism, the precursor to colonial development. Prior to the epidemic in Busoga, the focus of colonial medicine had been to keep whites alive in Africa. According to the logic of constructive imperialism, colonialism was to organize and train African labor to make colonies economically profitable. In the face of an indigenous epidemic in Uganda, a first step in this policy meant colonial science shifting its aims for the first time to keeping Africans alive and healthy.[2]

THE SCIENTIFIC SCRAMBLE FOR SLEEPING SICKNESS

The timing and drama of the epidemic in Uganda initiated a scientific scramble to understand and control sleeping sickness. In 1903 Albert Cook, a missionary doctor working in the epidemic area was among the first to help alert the colonial administration to the existence of a problem, noted that scientists from all over Africa and Europe were converging on the epidemic and that Uganda had become "the happy hunting ground for scientists."[3] Involvement with sleeping sickness research and control furthered individuals' careers, helped establish professions in biomedicine and the natural sciences, and served to carve out positions for scientists within the colonial state apparatus.

The British Foreign Office asked the Royal Society to send a commission of scientific inquiry to Uganda in 1902. The commission was made up of two

British scientists from Patrick Manson's London School of Tropical Medicine, George Low and Cuthbert Cristy, and an Italian student there, Aldo Castellani. A second Royal Society commission arrived in mid-1903 under the direction of the British army medical surgeon David Bruce.[4] Castellani observed trypanosomes in the cerebrospinal fluid of sleeping sickness cases in the Royal Society laboratory in Entebbe in 1903. At the same time Bruce, who in 1896 had made the tsetse-trypanosome connection in cattle, recognized the protozoa in human blood. They both reported back to the Royal Society concurrently that sleeping sickness was trypanosomiasis and that tsetse was a disease vector.

A scientist's discovery of a part of a disease epidemiology was a means to professional fame and position in medical schools, schools of tropical medicine, and the government. Conclusions by Castellani and Bruce about the connections between sleeping sickness, trypanosomes, and tsetse flies drew scientists to study symptoms, drug treatments, prophylactics, hosts, and vectors. For sleeping sickness, research involved an unknown number of types of tsetse flies, a vast variety of possible game host species, livestock, trypanosome types, and fly habitat combinations of vegetation, soils, temperatures, and moisture. Douglas Haynes shows a dramatic increase at the end of the nineteenth century in the colonial demand for medical personnel that helped constitute and expand the medical profession with nearly 20 percent of British practitioners engaged in the colonies by 1900.[5] The inclusive entomology of sleeping sickness research and control extended this scientific boom to a broad range of new professions. In investigations of other so-called tropical diseases, there were limited moments for discovery of infectious organism, vectors of transmission, and drug cure. In contrast trypanosomiasis offered botanists, entomologists, geologists, zoologists, game-control officers, medical doctors, medical researchers, and colonial disease control policy makers and enforcers a broad range of opportunities for employment and professional success.

Professional rewards accrued to those who contributed to the knowledge and therefore to the power of tropical medicine. Patrick Manson, Robert Koch, David Bruce, David Nabarro, Aldo Castellani, and Charles Swynnerton are examples of the opportunities within sleeping sickness science for rapidly gaining or keeping political and professional power. Koch's work with sleeping sickness drug cures furthered his already prominent career and influence. Nabarro became a prominent professor of pathology in England.[6] Castellani, a young student researcher when he arrived in Uganda in 1902, went on to become head of Italian army medical services in the 1930s, was knighted in England, and ennobled in Italy.[7]

After the discovery of sleeping sickness, scientists drew together the historical narrative of scientific progress. British doctors had been describing sleeping sickness since the mid-eighteenth century in West Africa as "Sleepy Distemper" and "Negro Lethargy."[8] Thomas Winterbottom observed a symptom of sleeping sickness, swollen neck glands, subsequently known as "Winterbottom's sign" in 1803. Nineteenth-century Trypanosome Fever had been sleeping sickness. Castellani's trypanosoma matched those first observed by R. M. Forde, a British army surgeon, in the blood of an African in the Gambia in 1901 (thus the nomenclature of *trypanosoma gambiense*).[9]

The trypanosome link between human sleeping sickness and nagana also brought scientific attention to bear on tsetse fly. Prior to 1903, Westerners were interested in tsetse as a killer of cattle and horses. This connection was well-established in Western sources since the mid-nineteenth century. European settlers and hunters commented on flies destructive to cattle, horses, and oxen beginning in the early nineteenth century as they pushed north across the Vaal river from South Africa.[10] In 1858 David Livingston published an article on the tsetse threat to cattle, "Arsenic as a remedy for the tsetse bite," in the *British Medical Journal.*[11] Richard Burton described a cattle-killing fly in Unyamwezi in his 1860 book, *The Lake Regions of Central Africa.*[12] In 1880 Griffith Evans connected trypanosomes to a cattle and horse disease in India known as "surra." In 1896 David Bruce found trypanosomes in the blood of cattle suffering from a cattle disease in Natal and identified tsetse as a vector of the disease-causing trypanosomes. Bruce named the cattle disease *nagana*, supposedly a Zulu word for a state of depressed spirits, and identified game as a trypanosome reservoir.[13]

The discoveries in Uganda made the particular entomology of tsetse species important to human disease control. In 1903 Ernest Austin listed nine species of tsetse in the first comprehensive monograph on tsetse flies based on the collection in the British Museum.[14] Between 1903 and 1913, Western scientists named 10 new species or subspecies of tsetse from Africa and, between 1920 and 1933, six more.[15] With British sleeping sickness control based on understanding tsetse behavior and hosts and the destruction of tsetse habitat, the epidemiology of sleeping sickness expanded to include entomology, botany, and zoology.

IMAGES OF ORDER AND TROPICAL LUXURIANCE

The Busoga epidemic occurred in a tropical context. Western images of tropical nature and disease juxtaposed modernity with nature and the primitive. Nancy Stepan centers nineteenth-century images of tropical nature in discourses about evolution, race, culture, and environment. She argues Westerners represented tropical nature and tropical people as both symbols of exotic paradise and of a sinister prehistory of unrestrained nature and people. Miasma theory and tropical disease emerging as a distinct field of study reflected the dark side of the tropics.[16] Literature about the tropics was extremely popular in Europe and North America and evinced a growing reliance on the language of natural science. The process of identifying, defining, and categorizing tropical phenomena informed Western ideas about Africans, nature, and disease.

Uganda is an important African variation on Stepan's arguments about the meanings of tropical nature. Works about Uganda, and particularly the kingdom of Buganda, published in Europe from the 1860s through the early twentieth century assigned a distinctive set of environmental meanings to the area. European travelers, missionaries, and colonial officers focused on the kingdom of Buganda as an African anomaly—a well organized and affluent political state—an example of African economic and cultural potential. Texts depict the kingdom of Buganda as relatively civilized under cruel but effective state control and as rich with natural resources. At the same time, texts represent the hothouse luxuriance of nature in Uganda as threatening human health and productivity.

Because of the wealth, political order, and perceived productive potential of Buganda, early colonial literature was extensive and important in guiding colonial intervention. Writers were often self-referential. Western explorer-scientists, missionaries, employees of the Imperial British East Africa Company, and early colonial administrators read published accounts of Uganda as guides to their travels and work and responded to these works in their own memoirs. Gerald Portal, a colonial negotiator in Buganda in 1893, mentions the writings of John Speke, Henry Stanley, Emin Pasha, and missionaries in his memoirs.[17] F. D. Lugard carried Speke's 1864 *Journal of the Discovery of the Source of the Nile* with him to help him in IBEAC negotiations with the Bugandan state from 1890 to 1893.[18] The Protestant Bishop Alfred R. Tucker wrote in 1908 that so much had already been written on Uganda, that it was difficult for him to say anything new.[19] This historiographically formed Uganda dominated twentieth-century British colonial officials' views. Not only was the response of British scientists and administrators in Uganda to sleeping sickness shaped by a textually produced Uganda, but Western readers came to view sleeping sickness control policies through the lens these publications provided.

John Speke and James Grant, two of the most influential East African explorers, visited Uganda in 1862 trying to find the source of the Nile River. Speke, Grant, and Chaille-Long (who came on a mission in 1875) gave detailed attention in their travelogues to the kingdom of Buganda, each devoting over 100 pages to its history and characteristics.[20] Henry Stanley's visit in 1875, his subsequent call to missionize, and the attention surrounding the 1888 Emin Pasha rescue expedition generated colonial interest and competition over the area to the north of Lake Victoria. Most of volume 1 of Stanley's *Through the Dark Continent* (1878) deals with Buganda and neighboring kingdoms. These explorers' testimonies fueled the debate over the "Uganda Question" in the British parliament and press in the early 1890s—a major focus of the imperialist versus anti-imperialist debate.[21]

The British understanding of Buganda as a combination of political order and environmental affluence was a predictable outcome of a powerful literary tradition. In 1894 the Christian Mission Society (CMS) missionary R. P. Ashe explicitly wrote of his agreement with previous literary descriptions; he began with Speke's portrayal of Uganda as "a striking contrast to the surrounding tribes; and though a land where the direct cruelty and most callous indifference to human life or human suffering prevailed, yet not wanting in a certain kind of civilization of its own."[22] Twentieth-century colonialists followed a path formed by nineteenth-century travel writers who had repeatedly praised the Ganda as intelligent, industrious, and organized. Harry Johnston, the British Special Commissioner in Uganda and architect of the Uganda Agreement in 1900 between Britain and the Ganda elite, asked readers of his two volume *The Uganda Protectorate* (1902) to imagine Uganda as "a black travesty" of an early Victorian painting, "'The Plains of Heaven,' wherein the Ganda move about like saints in long trailing garments. At great assemblies, in marketplaces, before the churches or law courts, or the residences of chiefs."[23]

Western discussions about the modern and the primitive linked morality and hygiene, civilization and attention to bodily order. In 1864 Grant wrote that Ganda homes "were superior to any we had met with in Africa—loftier, better constructed and more cleanly."[24] People wore shoes and clean clothes, made either of well-crafted bark-cloth or imported cotton: "There is scarcely any Muganda now so poor but that he cannot afford to wear a long trailing shirt of white cotton or linen."[25] Alluding to racist views of blacks and with the desire to differentiate Ganda from other Africans, Stanley wrote, "You must discard from your mind the . . . maudlin, filthy negro" and imagine "a cleanly decent creature."[26] In 1911 John Roscoe, another CMS missionary, wrote that "the Baganda belong to the great Bantu family, and are perhaps the most advanced and cultured tribe of that family."[27] British travelers Cherry Kearton and James Barnes wrote in 1915, "The Buganda are the most intelligent, wealthy, and industrious, the best looking, and the most polite of the many tribes with whom we came in contact."[28] Such opinions implied that the Ganda were then worthy of colonial investment.

Western reports connected material wealth and a flourishing economy with state control of an industrious work force. In 1878 the Austrian-born, Egyptian governor of Equatoria, Emin Pasha, wrote, "The Waganda and the Wanyoro have brought commerce to a more advanced state of development, corresponding to their higher civilization."[29] From the royal palaces to the family farms, images paired political order with abundance. State control of social behavior through a rigid status system channeled Ganda "natural" work ethic into agricultural and craft production. Indeed, according to Stanley, the desire to work "appears to be infused into their veins,"[30] and Bishop Tucker was "not at all sure that the Englishman is more ready to work."[31] Tucker complimented Ganda building techniques, legal and military organization, state administration, agricultural skills, and ironwork, comparing them favorably with the British: "Their forgings of knife blades being quite equal if not superior to the forgings of Sheffield."[32] Though reports of opulence and an excess of food and material wealth among the Ganda elite also associated the

Bugandan king (the Kabaka) and his court with Western images of decadent feudal absolutism, colonial literature emphasized that food was plentiful for all, and "real poverty did not exist."[33]

Writers cited Ganda control of the natural environment as the underlying cause of abundance and fertility. The colonial officer Gerald Portal wrote that the Ganda "keep the banana plantations in beautiful order, free from weeds, cutting away the decaying leaves, plucking the fruit at the right moment, and so forth."[34] Colonial authors such as Lord Lugard depicted Ganda as exploiting environmental opportunities, taking advantage of their great lumber forests, for example, to build canoes, houses, and bark-cloth garments, and plant trees.[35] Emin Pasha promoted Buganda by depicting it as an ideal vision of productivity: "On all the hills which we subsequently passed people were industriously employed, new fields and plantations were springing into existence, and bonfires of plucked-up grass sent forth clouds of smoke and the smell of burning. The women were busy digging in the fields, planting sweet potatoes or plucking up the grass; the men were building houses or enlarging and clearing roads, which here leads evenly over firm ferruginous clay."[36] Harry Johnston's depiction of the Buganda capital at Mengo emphasized his admiration of the city's domesticated and genteel urban space with cleanly defined private property: "Reed fences enclose the ground on either side of the broad red road. Behind these reed fences are numerous courtyards in which bananas grow. Everything bears a neat, swept-up appearance, and the handsome trees and general richness of vegetation round the dwellings make it a city of gardens."[37] Western authors linked Ganda agricultural productivity and economic prosperity to control over nature by noting the similarities between Ganda and British uses of roadways, fences, and hedges. Johnston described constructions of roads and paths crossing over dikes, bridges, and causeways, "running for miles in the most delightful shade between high hedges of cultivated dracaenas or other large-foliaged plants."[38]

While European observers praised the Ganda for effectively exploiting their natural resources, an emphasis on natural luxuriance brought that very same control of nature into question. Images of tropical exuberance undermined Ganda productive agency. Stanley, whose enthusiasm reflected his imperial agenda, wrote of "luxuriant plenty, wondrous greenness of the banana fronds, the bulk and number of the fruit, the fatness of the soil and its inexhaustible fertility, the perpetual spring-like verdure of the vegetation."[39] European observers consistently hinted at the idea that environmental fertility posed the problem of being a disincentive for African hard work: "In Uganda proper, owing to the abundant rainfall, there is food for all in limitless quantities, and with a minimum of labor, as the endless banana plantations require little or no attention, and the banana plant is capable of renewing itself when the parent tree dies."[40] "It was a perfect paradise for negroes: as fast as they sowed, they were sure of a crop without much trouble."[41] "They have little or nothing to do for their daily food, as the rich soil yields of itself all that is wanted in this way."[42] While the British imagined the Ganda as a stable and industrious workforce in control of their environments, British discussions of nature gave credit to forces beyond the control of the Ganda farmer and state.

In colonial texts, natural luxuriance allowed African socioeconomic order, but also sometimes threatened that order, and was sometimes threatened by it. In descriptions of Uganda, nature threatened human order: "The pleasant impression is shaken on closer inspection by the discovery that, except where its place is taken by the banana gardens, this wealth of verdure consists, not of growing crops and luxuriant cultivation, but of an impervious tangle of tall elephant grass whose close-growing cane-like stems offer an effective barrier to the comfortable progress of almost any living creature."[43] Johnston ends his "The Plains of Heaven" analogy with an image of nature at least equal to human action: "The fantastic vegetation of ultra-tropical richness with its palms and bananas, the gleaming water of lake, inlet, or swamp, the red roads, intensely green grass, brilliantly coloured flowers, and amidst this riot of colour and form the thousands of moving figures."[44] For the Western traveler in Buganda and the Western reader, just beyond human order lurked the "riot" of nature: "On the outskirts of nearly every village, banana plants may be seen carrying on an unequal struggle for life with the overpowering grass."[45] The landscape aesthetic contrasting productive order with natural luxuriance in Buganda created a rhetorical need for some system to bring a sense of order to nature.

Images of Uganda as tropical nature also linked luxuriance to decay and sickness. Portal imagined any Westerner would travel in Buganda "with a sigh of perplexity as he passes from the tangled waste through the carefully-tended and fruit-laden banana grove, from the bright air of the hillside to the death dealing miasma of the foetid swamp."[46] Miasma theory was a nineteenth-century explanation of disease as emanating from the ground in the form of gases, exacerbated by heat and carried by wind. These gases led to white deaths.[47] For Chaille-Long miasma meant Uganda was "but nothing—absolutely nothing—of that grand magnificent spectacle depicted by the pens of more enthusiastic travelers, who would make, to willing readers, a paradise of Africa, which in reality is, and must ever be a grave-yard to Europeans."[48] "Here, indeed," he emphasized, "is the Africa of my boyish Fancy! a hell on earth, whose rich vegetation and flowers, like the upas tree, breathe poison and death."[49] The utopia represented by the botanical garden was this hell brought to scientific order.

The connection between luxuriant nature and disease remained even after colonial science had discredited miasma theory. In 1926 Herbert Gresford, the Bishop of Kampala in the 1920s, depicted "beautiful evergreen forests" in Uganda as treacherous to humans in their deceptive beauty:

You have only to sit alone on the verandah in the short African twilight, when the mind is receptive to impressions, to feel this ominous unaccountable shadow that preys upon life. It is not difficult then to imagine how in beautiful evergreen forests, below the rank mass of undergrowth, something real and sinister is urging those cruel, tightly-clinging creepers to choke slowly and surely the life out of trees . . . that in this chill, penetrating miasma rising from the swamps is something heavy and malevolent. . . . [50]

Colonial reports of the 1902 sleeping sickness epidemic reinforced these images of Ugandan nature as diseased and threatening.

Colonialists used scientific nomenclature, at first descriptively, then in practice, to sort out the "impervious tangle" of nature in Uganda. Recent theorists of colonial travel writing such as Mary Louise Pratt have noted how natural science tends to produce literary visions which "conceived of the world as a chaos out of which scientists produced an order."[51] The Linnean descriptive system of nature classification was a transformative vehicle for Western scientific power. Carolus Linnaeus was an eighteenth-century Swedish botanist and taxonomist considered the originator of the modern scientific nomenclature of plant and animals with the publication of *Systema naturae* (1735) and *Genera plantarum* (1737). Students of Linnaeus fanned out across "unknown" areas of Africa, Asia, the Americas, and the Pacific, naming and categorizing unknown species of plants and animals.[52] As Pratt demonstrates, this process presented itself as nonimperial, "claiming no transformative power whatsoever."[53] In the context of colonial travel writing about Africa, in this use of scientific nomenclature as anti-conquest, the naturalist, "naturalizes the bourgeois European's own global presence and authority."[54]

The language of scientific objectivity was important to the identity and authority of explorers such as Grant, Speke, and Stanley, who represented themselves through their writings as explorer-scientists, where exploration permitted the opportunity for scientific discovery. Scientific nomenclature in Uganda was a colonial means toward legitimizing the appropriation of resources placed outside Buganda state control. Speke, for example, wrote of Uganda's "streaky argillaceous sandstones."[55] Stanley included alongside his romantic praise of Ganda forests, "whose meeting tops create night, into leafy abysms," lists of tree and plant species: "gigantic sycamore, towering mvule, and branchy gum."[56]

There were also renowned scientist-explorers such as Franz Stuhlman, Oscar Baumann, and Paul Kollman who emphasized that the value of their explorations of the Great Lakes region was in their scientific training. The appendixes of Baumann's 1894 travelogue included sections on stones, plants, mollusks, insects, cattle, linguistics, and African skull measurements.[57] Missionaries were no less inclined to scientific descriptions of Ugandan environments. CMS missionary Mackay mentioned "kaolin—a stratum of white clay below the red clay."[58] By the turn of the century, scientific references had become increasingly important to establishing both the legitimacy of the colonial text and the integrity of its author, and colonial control over African nature.

One consequence of such natural-science rhetoric was that European observers of nature could relegate Africans to the margins and de-emphasize both African control of the environment and Africans' occupation of their own lands:

As we marched between banana groves and huts, the country looked like a garden, Mother Nature having everywhere filled up the gaps left by man with glorious grass vegetation and graceful slender trees. Impenetrable thickets at times fringed the road, and one's eye became perfectly dazzled by the sight of so many shapes and colours. The odour of Umbelliferae mingled with the almost overpowering scent of a Liliaceous plant. Gigantic trees waved their lofty crowns in the sunlight, and below them, in the deep cool shade, climbing plants of every kind were interwoven. Elegant palm bushes shared the ground with splendid ferns (Asplenium), and parasitic plants, probably Angraecum and Platycerium, grew on the branches of sycamores and Spathodeas, so high up they were beyond reach.

Thus, artificial and natural gardens constantly alternated, though the former, consisting of bananas and sweet potatoes, could not possibly vie with the latter either in picturesque beauty or variety of species. This is indeed a beautiful, well-favoured land, with its red soil, its green gardens, its lofty mountains, and its dark snug valleys. Nature has profusely lavished her charms, and man alone destroys the harmony of these scenes.[59]

In this passage, vegetation not only inhabits and structures space, but is personified in favorable contrast to Africans. In Emin Pasha's prose, descriptions of nature overwhelm human actions. The author mentions Ugandans only as disturbances to an at once scientific and metaphysical environment.

Emin Pasha's critique of Africans' disrupting the "natural gardens" of Uganda reinforces Richard Grove's argument of the importance of Western idea of the botanical garden to colonialism. European Romanticism represented the nonurban redemptive potential of nature as paradise.[60] Thus, early colonialist-scientists saw botanical and taxonomic work as a retreat from social corruption and personal disappointments. According to Richard Grove, "By preventing alteration to the 'naturalness' of an island in terms of species, forest, climate, organized according to 'natural laws', the virtues of a non-European and non-corrupt Utopia could be maintained."[61] Beyond this general assessment of the meaning of botany and the botanical garden as a way to order and display (control) the unknown, when applied to African settings, it served to position African farmers and pastoralists acting on their environments as threats to natural harmony.

In Uganda, colonial officials drew on the idea of the botanical garden and their interest in natural science in formulating environmental interventions. Hesketh Bell, the governor of Uganda from 1905 to 1909, who first implemented sleeping sickness control policies, commented on how Entebbe had been built as a garden-city;[62] Alexander Whyte, a colonial officer in the 1890s, created the colonial station there as a botanical garden.[63] Whyte limited the clearing of trees and carefully located buildings to esthetically both fit into the garden landscape and provide the best views of Lake Victoria and Ugandan vegetation. In his memoirs, Bell presents gardening as an analogy to colonial governing. He relates a statement made to him by a British army lieutenant in Uganda: "Well, sir, if it is delightful to lay out a garden, how glorious it must be to lay out a protectorate!"[64] Colonial administrators had the power to join scientific understandings of nature with policy. In Uganda, Governor Bell and medical officer A. D. P. Hodges formulated and implemented the first colonial sleeping sickness policies beginning in 1906. They based policy on the epidemiological conclusions of Royal Society reports. Bell's interest in natural science made him receptive to policies of environmental intervention. With his mandate to establish colonial structures in Uganda and his alliance with scientists, Bell experimented with interventionist environmental policies.[65] The ideas of idealized nature and natural luxuriance were important contexts for the forms sleeping sickness control would take in Uganda.

DISEASE AND THE MASCULINIZATION OF COLONIAL SCIENCE

Western images of sleeping sickness and tsetse lent certain meanings to Ugandan environments and a new kind of heroics to colonial actions and colonial science. The scramble to understand and control tropical diseases began what David Arnold calls "the heroic age of medical intervention."[66] The perceived heroics of colonial science lent it cultural and political power, and helped propel the language and methods of science to the center of modern colonialism. The heroics of science represented a new kind of masculinity. Historians and cultural studies theorists have written about how Western science constructed gender, and about how important colonial sites as meeting grounds between the modern and the primitive were for Western understandings of race and gender.[67] Warwick Anderson writes that tropical colonies "presented both a special resource for white male self-fashioning and its testing ground."[68] But while these authors examine how scientists imagine race and gender, they do not look at how colonial settings masculinized scientists and how in turn the language and methods of science lent a masculine heroic legitimacy to all colonial interventions.[69]

Images of Victorian scientists epitomized the late-nineteenth-century idea of overcivilization that Anderson explains as mental work at the expense of body work, lacking aggression, masculinity, athletics, and virility.[70] Masculine critiques of science as feminized and overcivilized undermined its cultural and political power. But colonial scientists working in diseased places with primitive people reassumed manly qualities while avoiding the taint of the excesses of brutality faced by colonial soldiers. Popular texts promoted colonial scientists, and they promoted themselves, as aggressive in the pursuit of knowledge, as virile and athletic in moving through Africa to defend Africans from disease and environmental disorder.

The progress of sleeping sickness research and control was followed closely in Western newspapers and professional science journals beginning in 1902 as heroic and humanitarian. Such prominent scientists and officials involved with sleeping sickness as David Bruce, Robert Koch, Hesketh Bell, David Nabarro, and Aldo Castellani published pieces in the *Times* and in the popular press throughout Europe, Africa, and the United States; innumerable articles monitored their work, recommendations, and conferences in these years.[71] Hesketh Bell, the governor of Uganda, received public financial support for sleeping sickness control in Uganda by asking for donations in a *Times* article in April 1908.[72]

The *Times* gave particular attention to the controversy over the discovery of sleeping sickness and devoted space whenever scientists proffered claims of a cure. Between 1907 and 1913 the scientific community in Europe argued extensively in print whether the British David Bruce or the Italian Aldo Castellani discovered of the cause of sleeping sickness. The *Times* published letters to the editor on the subject from their supporters between 1907 and 1913, furthering European public interest in and acceptance of the significance of scientific activities in Africa.[73]

Douglas Haynes argues the importance of British medical publications in linking British medicine and imperialism and in presenting medicine as "a force of progress and symbol of modernity." *Lancet* and the *British Medical Journal* followed colonial activities closely. Patrick Manson, director of the London School of Tropical Medicine and the first medical advisor to the Colonial Office in 1897, aggressively worked to generate publicity about colonial medical discoveries. By emphasizing that sleeping sickness might be a threat to India, Manson contributed to a climate of anxiety about disease in the empire that enhanced the reputation and political power of scientists.[74]

Beginning after World War I, press coverage reflected further concerns over the globalization of sleeping sickness, reporting suspected cases throughout Europe, from Finland to France to Russia, as well as in New Zealand and Paraguay. The *Times* covered suspected outbreaks of sleeping sickness in Hungary in 1917 and in Lincolnshire in 1920.[75] These cases were mostly medical misdiagnoses. They expressed the heightened Western anxiety about disease in light of the health issues facing Europe after World War I and the influenza pandemic of 1918.

Western doctors' diagnoses of sleeping sickness outside Africa, press decisions to follow Western scientists' struggles with the tropical infection so closely, and the extent of scientific and popular publishing about sleeping sickness are indicators of the cultural and professional importance of sleeping sickness. Sleeping sickness and tsetse infused existing science publications with new significance and helped generate an explosion of new publishing venues for scientists. Between 1903 and 1963, scientific British and British colonial journals from *Experimental Parasitology* and the *Journal of Natural History*, to *Medical History* and *Veterinary Research* published articles on sleeping sickness and tsetse.

Since the mid-nineteenth century, colonial authors presented tsetse flies as a test of Europeans' mettle and a challenge to European colonization, imbuing colonial actions with a sense of heroic sacrifice and danger. David Livingstone emphasized the danger of tsetse and travel in Africa in 1857 in *Missionary Travels and Researches in South Africa*. The publishers of this influential and widely sold book put a drawing of a tsetse fly on the title page and other drawings in the text of tsetse—life-sized, magnified, and focusing on the proboscis. Livingston gave detailed descriptions of the effects of tsetse and infested areas.[76]

Western popular literature represented tsetse as an environmental barrier to colonization. David Livingstone wrote that the presence of tsetse indicated a distinct divide in African landscapes: Europeans could not live where there were tsetse.[77] In H. Rider Haggard's popular *King Solomon's Mines*, first published in 1885, tsetse were one of the series of barriers the group of white explorers pass through on their way to the mines.[78] Paul du Chaillu, in an 1869 book aimed specifically at young readers, *Wild Life Under The Equator*, included a chapter on the torments of various types of flies he encountered during his travels in Africa, including the "tsetche."[79] Chaillu recounted tsetse as "savage" and "dreaded" and that their bite was "quite as painful as a scorpion."[80]

The cultural meaning of flies became all the more powerful after scientists made the connection between tsetse and sleeping sickness gave tsetse a scientifically determined relationship to death. In *The Bonds of Africa: Impressions of Travel and Sport from Cape Town to Cairo 1902–1912*, Owen Letcher titled his chapter on Uganda, "The Devil in God's Garden." Letcher wrote of the epidemic as "a great cloud of death." He concluded, "It seems as though the plagues of the Pharaohs have hastened down the Nile to stay the advance of modern days, and well they have succeeded."[81] Sleeping sickness was a literary personification of the threat of tropical Africa. In the beginning chapter of *Alone in the Sleeping-Sickness Country*, Felix Oswald recalled village ruins and emaciated Africans in Kavirondo just waiting to die. He wrote of himself being bitten by tsetse: "It was not until two months after my return to England that I could be sure that I was not infected."[82] Caroline Kirkland ended her chapter on sleeping sickness from the 1908 travelogue, *Some African Highways: A Journey of Two American Women to Uganda and the Transvaal*, with a description of going to bed at night in Entebbe while pondering the sleeping sickness epidemic: "The night is palpable, suffocating, appalling, and filled with a nameless horror which is quite indescribable."[83]

The presence of tsetse and therefore of sleeping sickness invigorated travel in Africa as life threatening, and colonial authors used them to promote the drama of colonialism. Authors wrote of the devastation, deaths, depopulated lands, and empty harbors caused by sleeping sickness. Kirkland describes the history of the epidemic in Uganda, the number of deaths, and deserted villages.[84] In the introduction of *Adventures in Africa under the British, Belgian and Portuguese Flags*, J. B. Thornhill assured readers that he had included in his book "a description of that terrible scourge."[85] Alfred Tucker discussed the particulars of sleeping sickness in a chapter entitled "Sunshine and Shadow."[86] In *Through Uganda to Mount Elgon*, J. B. Purvis juxtaposes the beauty of Uganda and the dangers of sleeping sickness in the chapter, "The Lake Victoria: Its Surroundings and Scourge."[87]

These descriptions used sleeping sickness to emphasize both the overwhelming and corrupt power of nature in Africa and the romance of being in such dangerous places: "There is something particularly sinister in this slow, stealthy, irresistible approach of death, whose course no known remedy can stay or alter."[88] Sleeping sickness and tsetse became emblematic of the African colonial experience.

The imagining of the sleeping sickness scientist as hero was pervasive in popular literature. Texts about colonial scientists depicted them risking the dangers of trypanosomiasis not for their own profit and thrill as with white hunters but for the advancement of science and the protection of African lives. By taking up the challenge of tropical disease, colonial science reemphasized Africa as a threat and scientists as adventurers on the frontiers of colonization. Many of the medical doctors and scientists involved with sleeping sickness published their own autobiographies and had biographies written about them (see figure 2.1). These works are noncritical, presenting the scientists as inspirational figures of altruism and sacrifice. Stories of sleeping sickness research and control presented colonial scientists as working at great risk but never shirking their responsibilities. K. C. Willet, for example, while discussing the need to establish local African confidence in scientific medical treatment, writes that doctors Corson and Fairbairn first infected themselves with trypanosomes to show local people their good intentions.[89] In *Man Against Tsetse*, John McKelvey employs the quote, "You tell me to sit quiet," to illustrate the indignation sleeping sickness scientists felt in Africa when colonial bureaucracy or politics hampered their work.[90] The depiction of the white doctor in Africa reified Africa as a place of danger and evil and Africans as primitive other, and placed doctors as defending order from chaos.[91] Tsetse and sleeping sickness were powerful and foundational examples of this cultural process.

Winston Churchill's book, *My African Journey* (1908), was a dramatic and overt example of the linking of popular literature, colonial science, and colonial politics. Churchill, as an elite British politician and state official, presented sleeping sickness and the potential of Western science as a justification and necessity for British colonial rule in Uganda. Churchill wrote that "a new

Figure 2.1
Publications on Scientists as Heroes in Africa

	Includes Discussion of Sleeping Sickness
Autobiography:	
Ronald Ross, *Memoirs* (London, 1923)	yes
Paul White, *Doctor in Tanganyika* (series) (London, 1944)	yes
Albert Cook, *Uganda Memories* (Kampala, 1945)	yes
James McCord, *My Patients Were Zulus* (London, 1946)	no
Albert Schweitzer, *On the Edge of the Primeval Forest* (London, 1948)	yes
Werner Junge, *African Jungle Doctor* (London, 1952)	no
M. Vane, *Black and White Medicine* (London, 1957)	yes
Aldo Castellani, *Microbes, Men and Monarchs: A Doctor in Many Lands* (London, 1960)	yes
Alfred Merriweather, *Desert Doctor: Medicine and Evangelism in the Kalahari Desert* (London, 1964)	no
Leader Stirling, *Tanzanian Doctor* (with an introduction by Julius Nyerere) (London, 1977)	no
Louise Jilejk-Aall, *Call Mama Doctor: African Notes of a Young Woman Doctor* (London, 1980)	no
W. E. Davis, *Caring and Curing in Congo and Kentucky* (North Middletown, 1984)	yes
Biography:	
E. Ray Lankester, *The Kingdom of Man* (London, 1907)	yes
Paul De Kruif, *Microbe Hunters* (New York, 1926)	yes
P. H. Manson-Bahr, *The Life and Work of Sir Patrick Manson* (New York, 1927)	yes
Edith Hutchings, *The Medicine Man: Stories from Medical Missions in India, China, Africa, and Madagascar* (London, 1927)	no
R. L. Megroz, *Ronald Ross: Discoverer and Creator* (London, 1931)	yes
Paul De Kruif, *Men Against Death* (New York, 1932)	no
P. F. Russell, *Man's Mastery of Malaria* (London, 1953)	no
M. Gelfand, *Tropical Victory* (London, 1953)	yes
Joyce Reason, *Safety Last* (London, 1954)	no
Brian O'Brien, *That Good Physician* (London, 1962)	yes
Berton Roueche, *Annals of Epidemiology* (Boston, 1967)	no
A. C. and P. Clegg, *Man Against Disease* (London, 1973)	yes
J. Brabazon, *Albert Schweitzer* (New York, 1975)	yes
M. Gelfand, *A Service to the Sick* (Gwelo, 1976)	no
W. D. Foster, *Sir Albert Cook* (London, 1978)	yes
Oliver Ransford, *Bid the Sickness Cease: Disease in the History of Black Africa* (London, 1983)	yes
Sleeping Sickness Specific:	
T. A. M. Nash, *Africa's Bane: The Tsetse Fly* (London, 1969)	yes
John McKelvey, *Man Against Tsetse: Struggle for Africa* (Ithaca, 1973)	yes

opponent has appeared and will not be denied. Uganda is defended by its insects."[92] Churchill described sleeping sickness as a "terrible shadow" darkening the protectorate. In Churchill's eight-page history of the discovery of the disease and early intervention, initially sleeping sickness resisted treatment and seemed "universally fatal": "It seemed certain that the entire population of the districts affected was doomed." But "the police of science" arrived in the persons of colonial officials such as David Bruce and Hesketh Bell, and "knowledge has accumulated." Churchill promised that currently control policies seemed to be working and "there must be no losing heart":[93]

The police of science, although arrived late on the scene of the tragedy, are now following many converging clues. Knowledge has accumulated. The humble black horse-fly—International Commissions discuss him round green tables, grave men peer patiently at him through microscopes, active officers scour Central Africa to plot him out on charts. A fine-spun net is being woven remorselessly around him.[94]

His conclusion to the chapter on Uganda was a dramatic presentation of the colonial alliance between science and imperialism:

But what an obligation, what a sacred duty is imposed upon Great Britain to enter the lists in person and to shield this trustful, docile, intelligent Baganda race from dangers which, whatever their cause, have synchronized with our arrival in their midst! And, meanwhile, let us be sure that order and science will conquer, and that in the end John Bull will be really master in his curious garden of sunshine and deadly nightshade.[95]

Churchill presented the scientific colonization of African disease as a British mission in Uganda. He justified British occupation by showing colonial officers involved not in militarily subjugating Africans but rather in mapping tsetse areas to save Africans from disease.

GANDA IMPERIAL INTERESTS

While scientists had increasing political and cultural power in the imperial metropole and in the colonies, Africans influenced Western images of Africa and the forms of colonial sleeping sickness research and control and their meanings for Europeans. Furthermore, African elite, fishers, and farmers understood colonial sleeping sickness control in their own political, economic, and environmental contexts. For example, in the late nineteenth and early twentieth centuries, the Ganda state promoted images of order and state power to outsiders. These images reinforced Ganda state abilities to avoid, or at least manage, foreign intervention in the area and effectively reinforced Ganda state and imperial power, all of which informed the history of British sleeping sickness control. Baganda exercised a great deal of power in controlling European access and influence to the north of Lake Victoria. Africans, in part, controlled what early European explorers and colonial representatives saw. In the nineteenth century, state officials met European travelers to Buganda at the borders, and the Buganda state monitored and controlled Westerners' movements for the duration of their visits. Officials timed foreign visitors' entry into the capital at Mengo, their travels on and around the lake, and their early visits to the Nile outlet in ways designed to promote images of Ganda power and affluence. The generosity and friendliness shown to European visitors served to control and direct attention to Ganda surpluses. John Speke reported that in 1862 he was not allowed to buy food by orders of the Kabaka, who instructed him and his entourage freely to take any food and supplies they wanted from fields or storage spaces.[96] By keeping Westerners on main roads and in organized canoe-fleets, the Buganda state presented strategic images of health, productivity, and order that promoted Buganda state legitimacy to the British.

European influence in Uganda began in the late 1870s with the arrival of Protestant and Catholic missionaries. Competition between Protestant, Catholic, and Muslim converts for power at the court of the Kabaka resulted in a period of civil war in Buganda in the 1880s and 1890s. Uganda became a British protectorate in 1890. In that year Frederick Lugard arrived in Buganda as a representative of the Imperial British East Africa Company (IBEAC). Lugard involved himself in court politics, allying with a faction of Christian chiefs against the Kabaka Mwanga. In 1899 the IBEAC-Christian alliance militarily overthrew Mwanga and installed the young Daudi Chwa as the new Kabaka. Three senior Christian chiefs who were regents for Daudi Chwa effectively ruled Buganda in his name.

At the same time British officials were consolidating power in Buganda through this alliance, British military forces were helping Buganda armies extend regional Ganda hegemony. Buganda was an aggressive imperial state with a long history of imperial expansions and contractions. Beginning in the early eighteenth century, Buganda armies frequently raided neighboring territories of Bunyoro to the northwest, Busoga to the east, and the Buvuma and Sesse island groups in northern Lake Victoria for slaves and cattle. Along with raiding, Buganda sought to establish tribute relations that would provide Buganda with regular gifts of food, slaves, and material goods and to expand the borders of Buganda proper.

The late nineteenth century was a time of Ganda military aggression against Banyoro, Basoga, and Bavuma, which would become centers of future colonial sleeping sickness control.[97] In the mid-1880s Bunyoro turned back an invading force of Ganda soldiers.[98] Historically, Buganda and Bunyoro competed for power in Busoga, raiding, demanding tribute, and intervening in Soga succession disputes. Through the nineteenth century, parts of southern Busoga were tributary possessions of Buganda, although random Ganda expeditions still raided for booty, and the Buganda military occasionally invaded to reaffirm Ganda dominance.[99] Ganda chiefs had authority over subject Busoga districts, and Soga chiefs were in attendance at the court of the Kabaka.[100]

Lake Victoria was an important route for Ganda trade and imperial expansion and would be a major focus of colonial sleeping sickness control. The Lake Victoria islands had symbolic, political, and economic importance for the Buganda state. Sesse islanders made up the bulk of the Ganda navy and provided canoes. In 1894 R. P. Ashe wrote, "Owners of these islands practically held all the water communications on the lake."[101] In 1878 a Ganda fleet invaded Ukerewe Island in the far southern lake, and other fleets of hundreds of Sesse canoes with Sesse crews were employed in Ganda attacks on Buvuma and Busoga.[102] During civil war in 1891–92, Protestant and Catholic chiefs competed for authority over the Sesses as vital locations for basing operations and providing manpower and material.[103] All the land between the Kabaka's palace and Lake Victoria was under the Kabaka's private control. This land represented direct access both to lake resources and trade and served as a convenient route of escape during political crises. During the War of Succession from 1889 to 1890, Kabaka Mwanga II fled the capital to the island of Bulingugwe. With Sesse islander support, he returned to the mainland and regained power.[104]

The economic and political importance of islander canoes and crews for Buganda was reflected in religious status. The Sesse Islands were known by the Ganda as the "Mother of the Gods." In Ganda theology, the primary deities were all originally from the Sesse Islands: the lake deity and god of plenty Mukasa, his father Musisi, grandfather Wanga, and brothers Wamala and the war god Kibuka.[105] The state temple of the lake deity Mukasa, one of the four primary state temples in the Buganda kingdom, was located on Bubembe Island in the Sesses. This temple was heavily subsidized by annual tribute from the Kabaka, and the temple priests had ritual control over all lake canoe traffic and over the war fleets. The primary ruler of the Sesses, the Gabunga, held a great deal of independent power. He was admiral of the Ganda navy, and the Kabaka appointed him from the Sesse-based Mamba clan.[106]

Islanders maintained a degree of political independence from the mainland that posed threats to Ganda authority. The Bavuma actively resisted Ganda expansion. Bavuma naval skills and resources helped defend them against their larger and more militarily powerful, land-based neighbor. A Ganda attack on Buvuma in 1875 failed miserably.[107] A Ganda raid on Kome Island in 1886 was likewise unsuccessful.[108] In 1893 the Bavuma refused to provide canoes to transport a Ganda army from Busoga to Buganda and raided Ganda islands to the west.

The Buganda state benefited geopolitically from British support of Buganda power against who the British imagined as Buganda's less civilized neighbors. Good relations between the IBEAC and the Ganda state after 1890 encouraged the British to view Buganda as a center of colonial potential and surrounding states and people as peripheral to a Ganda core. British-Ganda forces campaigned against neighboring Bunyoro, Busoga, and Buvuma who resisted the authority of the Buganda state. The political leader of Bunyoro, the Mukama Kabarega refused a British-brokered peace with Buganda, prompting Lugard to invade Bunyoro in 1893 with 15,000 troops, 14,000 of which were actually Ganda. A second invasion force in 1895 consisted of 20,000 Ganda along with six companies of Sudanese troops and British artillery. After continued resistance, Kabarega was captured by British-Ganda forces in 1899 and treated as occupied territory ruled from Buganda.

British officials were involved in military actions against the Bavuma as well. Henry Stanley participated in the failed Ganda attack of Buvuma in 1875.[109] The Bavuma refused to support the British-backed Christian chiefs in the civil wars during the 1880s and 1890s (they did not participate in these conflicts at all). In 1893 a joint Ganda-IBEAC force invaded Buvuma aided by the company's boats and machine guns and finally defeated the islanders.[110]

The Uganda Agreement of 1900 institutionalized the British-Ganda alliance and consolidated Ganda regional power. Bavuma and the Sesse Islands officially became part of Buganda while Busoga, Bunyoro, Toro, and Ankole were separate principalities administered by Ganda agents working for the British.[111] The Uganda Agreement awarded approximately 40 percent of what had been Bunyoro territory in 1890 to Buganda.[112] Sleeping sickness control actions in these areas were overt expressions of Ganda-British occupation.

British perceptions of relative Ganda wealth and productivity were connected to Ganda imperial tribute and conquest.[113] By promoting and confirming Western images of Buganda as productive, rich, clean, relatively "developed," and "civilized," Ganda helped place themselves above their neighbors in the eyes of the British. In doing so they enhanced their ability to dominate the area militarily, economically, and culturally. Thus in Roscoe's statement in his 1911 ethnography that the Buganda "don't travel far being surrounded by hostile tribes," readers understood "hostile tribes" as primitives who threatened Buganda order, not as people defending themselves from Ganda imperial aggression.[114]

British-Ganda military expeditions against the Nyoro and Bavuma gave the Buganda state further legitimacy in the eyes of colonial administrators as cooperative and effective. In turn, the British interpreted the alliance as Ganda support for the British colonial mission. From the perspective of the British, the Bavuma, Nyoro, and Soga proved themselves less advanced and less deserving of political autonomy and authority by resisting British-Ganda hegemony. British aid in extending Ganda authority was a part of both British and Ganda officials' understandings of the basis of cooperation between the two states. With the sleeping sickness epidemic of 1900, the logic of this cooperation was reinforced by observations of healthy Ganda environments relative to diseased neighboring environments.

Thus both the British and Ganda consolidated imperial authority when the British enforced sleeping sickness regulations outside Buganda through Ganda agents. The British administration explained the policy of appointing

Ganda administrators by pointing out the developmental advantages of "Ganda-ization" of rule by relatively advanced Ganda officials over the less developed as "a new generation of chiefs with ideas more enlightened and minds less besotted in youth with hemp and drink."[115] This policy, however, reflected how British power in the area depended on the aid and cooperation of the Buganda state. The Buganda state positioned itself in its support of sleeping sickness control so that it could not be easily sidestepped by the British. On the other hand, as I will explore in chapter 3, non-Ganda people understood Ganda-administered sleeping sickness depopulations in the context of their relationships with both Ganda and British imperial aggression.

Sleeping sickness was also a political disease since political conflict, economic disruptions, and demographic movements affected the expansion and contraction of tsetse and shifts between endemic and epidemic disease occurrences. Ganda and British-Ganda military aggression in the late nineteenth century created environmental and socioeconomic disruptions that lent momentum to cycles of disease and environmental crises including the expansion of tsetse and sleeping sickness. The Ganda religious center for Kaumpuli, the god of disease, was on the Bunyoro-Buganda border, an area regularly devastated by warfare and raiding.[116] The Ganda perceived the conflict-torn border area with Bunyoro as a place of desolation and pestilence. David Cohen argues that tribute raiding resulted either in regional adjustments of surplus production to meet tribute demands (as occurred in Busoga) and stable relationships with Ganda imperial rule, or socioeconomic devastation, depopulation, and the abandonment of productive environments.[117]

Rinderpest entered central Africa in 1891 devastating local economies and leading to the abandonment of pastures. Parts of Uganda, including Busoga, experienced drought beginning in 1898.[118] Military actions and the Uganda Agreement also generated increased regional migration and relocation. Refugees from war, disease, and land-ownership changes moved to the Lake Victoria shore to fish and trade. In areas of out-migration, the abandonment of farms and pastures led to the growth of brush and the expansion of tsetse. On the Lake Victoria shore in Busoga, an increase in refugees moving into and through this endemic sleeping sickness area might have brought more people in contact with tsetse and triggered the late-nineteenth-century epidemic.

The distribution of land and resources according to the Uganda Agreement lent further political meaning to colonial sleeping sickness controls. Within Buganda, according to the 1900 agreement, the Buganda state would collect and pay taxes to the British colonial administration and would enforce colonial regulations. In return, the Ganda elite maintained their positions and received land and salaries from the colonial administration. The Uganda Agreement divided land between direct colonial control and Buganda state control. The British negotiated colonial rule by assigning close to 9,000 square miles of land to the Kabaka, royal family members, and Ganda state officials as *mailo*, freehold lands.[119] According to this agreement, in Buganda the British administration could claim up to 9,000 square miles of uncultivated "waste" land and 1,500 square miles of forests as crown lands.[120] The agreement expanded Ganda territory and guaranteed the Ganda elite continued material wealth and political power. It confirmed de facto the cultivated holdings of the Ganda elite and allowed them to choose uncultivated land up to the total area agreed upon. Thus the Ganda elite came to possess both the best cultivated and uncultivated land.[121] This land deal was a central component of Ganda state cooperation with British colonial rule.

The distribution of private land and of authority over land through the preexisting structures of the Bugandan state set the stage for small-scale, peasant agricultural production of cotton and coffee cash crops. European plantation production remained minimal due to high transportation costs from Uganda to the coast, the global depression in the 1920s and 1930s, resistance from both the Buganda state and British administration in Uganda, and labor shortages due to farmer preferences to work land rented from Ganda elite. Farmers in Uganda increasingly used profits from the sale of cotton and coffee to buy small landholdings outright from Ganda elite. The elite sold off small holdings both to increase their immediate wealth and to increase their tax base since they also administered tax collection, in turn creating local-freehold, cash-crop farming.[122] The original 4,000 freeholds of the 1900 Uganda Agreement expanded by the 1950s to 50,000 freeholds.[123] In 1960 Uganda was the largest cotton producer in the British African territories and the largest coffee producer in the British commonwealth.[124]

The issue of the control of cash-cropped land generated tensions among Ganda elite, between Ganda elite and the British, and between farmers and government officials. Antigovernment riots (directed against both the British and Ganda administrations) in 1945 and 1949 involved popular concerns about state land alienation.[125] The political platforms of early nationalist parties in Uganda, such as the Bataka party founded in 1946 and the Uganda National Congress (UNC) founded in 1952, included opposition to the state acquisition of land. In Busoga the UNC joined resistance to state alienation of land with opposition to government-appointed chiefs.[126] Because sleeping sickness control involved the state alienation of land (if supposedly temporary), African elite and farmers understood disease control policies partially in the context of competition over land and resources. For example, the UNC agitated against state resettlement schemes of sleeping sickness areas in the 1950s as taking decisions about land distribution and control out of local hands and placing them in the hands of the government.

AFRICAN UNDERSTANDING OF ENVIRONMENT AND DISEASE

Farmers' and fishers' nineteenth-century relationships to environment and disease affected British visions and formed a lens through which local Africans viewed Anglo-Ganda sleeping sickness control. Baganda, Basoga, and Bavuma farmers' organization of human space and natural space usually centered around the banana garden. A homestead included a central compound, with structures for living, food storage, and livestock, surrounded by banana gardens and other cultivated areas, later including coffee and cotton plants as a main colonial cash crop. Banana trees could produce fruit year-round on the same land for 50 years or more and required little maintenance after the initial clearing and planting. Farmers often occupied the same homesteads for multiple generations.

Uncultivated space on the margins of homesteads demarcated the borders between homesteads, between villages, and between kingdoms. Networks of paths and roads wound through uncultivated areas. Local people regularly accessed what Gerald Portal described as "an effective barrier to the comfortable progress of almost any living creature."[127] Women and men entered the margins of homesteads and villages: to collect firewood, wood for building structures and canoes, and bark for bark-cloth; to hunt; to get water; and to gather other forest products. While border wilderness separated areas for farmers and fishers both literally and conceptually, forest resources were regularly accessed for daily household production.

The political economy of Buganda was structured around gender and class divisions of labor that supported a centralized state and imperial expansion. Nonelite women did a great deal of agricultural and domestic labor, but conventionally only men and royal women could hold land and political office. The Kabaka theoretically owned all land and distributed large estates with official titles. Except for clan-held lands, titles and holdings were nonhereditary and could be reclaimed at any time. The Ganda state system involved administrative landholding mobility as officials were regularly reassigned, promoted, and demoted.

The Ganda nonelite, known as *bakopi*, had legal access to land through cultivation rights called *kusenga* given by elite landholders in return for material tribute and labor. Material tribute was usually in the form of food, beer, or bark-cloth, and labor in the form of male military service or road upkeep.[128] The elite could not revoke land rights once they were granted; such rights were held in perpetuity or for as long as the elite family held title to the land and the farming family maintained residence. Landholders needed *bakopi* to meet the tribute required of them by their superiors, including the raising of troops. Elite upward mobility depended in part on material gifts to superiors and military success with *bakopi* troops. *Bakopi*, therefore, were in high demand.

The value of the *bakopi* was reflected in their rights to leave one *kusenga* relationship for another if dissatisfied with a patron.[129] Poorer, disliked, and downwardly mobile landholders found it more difficult to attract and keep farmers in *kusenga*. Rich and upwardly mobile titleholders could attract and keep people on their lands. Economic and political power resulted from retaining *bakopi* labor. The significance of *bakopi* labor is reflected in the Ganda saying, "One does not rule land, one rules people."[130] Farmers often followed landholders they had relationships with to new estates and administrative districts, and new officials evicted farmers to make room for themselves, their families, and the farmers following them from former assignments. The coming to power of a new Kabaka resulted in large-scale migrations of this kind, as did the new land assignments and political changes of the 1900 Uganda Agreement. The missionary Alfred Tucker observed that in 1901, "The whole population was in movement. Streams of men, women, and children going east with all their household goods, cattle, sheep, goats, and fowls, met similar streams going west. Evicted tenants from the north were able to greet their friends in a similar condition from the south."[131] *Kusenga* land rights were based on relationships to particular elite, not to the land itself. With the constant shuffling of state titles and *bakopi* residence choice, both elite and nonelite Ganda were geographically mobile.

Busoga and Bunyoro had systems, similar to Buganda, of state administrators whose reassignments caused farmer dislocation and land reallotment. But in both regions there was more lineage-group-based, hereditary land, and land tenure and access to pastures was more stable. In the various independent kingdoms of Busoga, family graves on homestead fields often held generations of ancestors.[132]

Bavuma and Sesse islanders did not have experience with state-ordered land allotment. Lineage groups controlled land, and land tenure was relatively stable. Even on the Sesse Islands, which were incorporated into the Ganda state in the nineteenth century, Ganda political rule did not bring about mobility as on the Ganda mainland. The Buganda state gained access to island labor and goods through tribute demanded of island clans. Islanders' experiences with dislocation were as victims of Ganda slave raids. Most recently in the British-Ganda attack on Buvuma in 1883, the Ganda took numerous Bavuma to the mainland as slaves.[133]

Land and labor relations at the turn of the century between farmers and African elite reflected local understandings of landscape and formed part of the context of people's responses to human sleeping sickness and to colonial disease controls. For the Ganda, the mobility *kusenga* afforded reinforced a precolonial disease control strategy of voluntary physical separation. In southern Uganda, colonial state and missionary reports and local people mentioned voluntary depopulation by Africans leaving diseased areas. Tsetse were endemic to the region, and local groups controlled tsetse environments through settlement patterns and by limiting contact with tsetse while hunting, fishing, and herding cattle. Although there is little evidence about precolonial Ganda understandings of disease, John Roscoe hints at the idea of human-disease vector separation in institutionalized Ganda medicine; Ganda priests took everyone away from an infected homestead. Reoccupation was forbidden until priests returned to purify the area.[134]

CONCLUSION

Turn-of-the-twentieth-century European observations about Uganda were continuations of long-standing discussions about Europe's relationship to Africa, about Ganda productivity, and the potential wealth of the colony. If travelers initially perceived Ugandan sicknesses and natural luxuriance as alienating, colonial science altered this view. Natural science and germ theory provided British colonizers with a language and a framework to understand environmental order as a way to promote health and profits of benefit to all.

Ganda elite and local farmers and fishers brought understandings of disease and environment to colonial relationships as well. Just as the conclusions and methods of scientists followed from the circumstances of their position in the West, perspectives emerged from within imperial, class and production relations, and local Africans' circumstances (such as how farmers managed their own gardens and fishers accessed the lake). Though the way in which the British imagined Uganda shaped early colonial actions and agendas, that the Ganda were actively involved in the manipulation of British images of Africa must be taken into account. The 1900 Uganda Agreement is one prime example of how Ganda elite exercised influence in the matter. The agreement reflected and recognized Buganda state authority and the belief of the British colonial administration that it was dependent on the maintenance and goodwill of that state's authority. The formulation of future colonial policies in Uganda would continue to reflect the extent to which popular images of Africa were integral to British colonization schemes. Likewise, political relationships between African elites and farmers and fishers, and the relationships of farmers and fishers to natural resources affected the ways in which local people understood sleeping sickness controls and formed a basis for their reactions to control regulations.

NOTES

1. Soff, "A History of Sleeping Sickness;" Langlands.
2. Worboys, "Comparative History," 91; Haynes, 470–472, 488.
3. Albert Cook, *Mengo Mission Notes*, (Albert Cook Library, 1903), quoted in Foster, 94.
4. Soff, "Sleeping Sickness Control."
5. Haynes, 471–472.
6. Soff, "A History of Sleeping Sickness," 87.
7. Ransford, 123–124.
8. The sickness was first named by British naval physician John Atkins in 1742 in West Africa.
9. McKelvey, 34, 43, 75–77; Nash, *Africa's Bane*, 25.
10. Nash, *Africa's Bane*, 22.
11. Livingston, "Arsenic as a Remedy," 360–361.
12. Burton, vol. 2, 18–19.

13. Nash, *Africa's Bane*, 24–25.

14. Ernest Edward Austin, *A Monograph of the Tsetse Flies Genus Glossina, Westwood Based on the Collection in the British Museum* (London, 1903); McKelvey, 12–18.

15. Ford, *African Ecology*, 42.

16. Stepan.

17. Portal, 180.

18. Lugard, 22.

19. Tucker, 91.

20. J. Speke; Grant; Chaille Long, *Central Africa: Naked Truths about Naked People* (New York, 1877).

21. D. A. Low, "British Public Opinion and the Uganda Question, October–December, 1892," *Uganda Journal* 18, 2(1954), 81–100; D. A. Low, *Buganda in Modern History* (Berkeley, 1971), 55–83.

22. R. P. Ashe, *Chronicles of Uganda* (London, 1894), 55.

23. Johnston, vol. 1, 104.

24. Grant, 216; J. Speke, 267.

25. Johnston, 104; also see Ashe, 56.

26. Stanley, vol. 1, 243.

27. Roscoe, 6.

28. Kearton and Barnes, 83–84.

29. Emin Pasha, *Emin Pasha in Central Africa: Being a Collection of His Letters and Journals* (London, 1888), 111.

30. Stanley, 243.

31. Tucker, 94.

32. Tucker, 95; Lugard, 1; Stanley, 243–261.

33. Roscoe, 12.

34. Portal, 199.

35. Lugard, 1.

36. Pasha, 125.

37. Johnston, 105–106.

38. Ibid., 68.

39. Stanley, 243.

40. J. F. Cunningham, *Uganda and Its People* (London, 1905), 302.

41. J. Speke, 258.

42. Mackay, 107.

43. Portal, 182.

44. Johnston, 104.

45. Henry E. Colville, *The Land of the Nile Springs* (London, 1895), 41.

46. Portal, 182.

47. Gallagher, 11–12.

48. Long, 125.

49. Ibid., 149.

50. Jones, 88.

51. Pratt, 30.

52. Ibid., 24–35.

53. Ibid., 38–39

54. Ibid., 28.

55. J. Speke, 257.

56. Stanley, 255.

57. Oscar Baumann, *Durch Massailand zur Nilquelle* (Berlin, 1894).

58. Mackay, 107.

59. Pasha, 125.

60. Grove, *Green Imperialism*, 232–236.

61. Ibid., 243, 240.

62. Hesketh Bell, *Glimpses of a Governor's Life* (London, 1946), 110–111.

63. Johnston, 118.

64. Lieutenant Fishbourne quoted in Bell, 124.

65. Grove, "Early Themes," 22.

66. David Arnold, "Introduction: Disease, Medicine, and Empire" in Arnold, *Imperial Medicine*, 21.

67. Levy; Cynthia Eagle Russett, *Sexual Science: The Victorian Construction of Womanhood* (Cambridge: Harvard University Press, 1989); Gail Bederman, *Manliness and Civilization: A Cultural History of Gender and Race in the United States, 1880–1917* (Chicago, 1995); Nupur Chadhuri and Margaret Strobel, eds., *Western Women and Imperialism: Complicity and Resistance* (Bloomington, 1992); Mrinalini Sinha, *Colonial Masculinities: The "Manly Englishman" and the "EffeminantBengali" in the Late Nineteenth Century* (Manchester, 1995).

68. W. Anderson, 1346.

69. An exception to this is Vaughan.

70. W. Anderson, 1348.

71. *Times* (London), November 7, 1903, 12 (Bruce); February 13, 1906, 4 (Koch); June 19, 1907, 7 (International Conference); December 24, 1906, 5a (Ross); January 10, 1907, 8c (Manson); March 14, 1908, 14b (Conference); July 23, 1908, 13f (Nabarro); April 17, 1909, 4f (Castellani). Coverage of sleeping sickness peaked in the *Times* from 1908 (over 50 articles) to 1913 (over 20 articles), and again in the mid-1920s (averaging over 20 articles annually).

72. Hesketh Bell, *Times* (London), April 9, 1908, 7.

73. *Times* (London), August 20, 1908, 7f; August 17, 1907, 4f; August 14, 1913, 4c; August 29, 1913, 3d; September 20, 1913, 5e.

74. Haynes, 480.

75. *Times* (London), July 3, 1917, 7c (Hungary); March 18, 1919, 9c (New York); July 16, 1920, 11f (Sweden); August 27, 1920, 7f (South Wales); May 6, 1920, 15f (Paris); March 29, 1920, 10c (Lincolnshire); February 13, 1920, 11f (Germany); November 29, 1920, 13f (Paraguay); February 16, 1923, 9g (Russia).

76. Livingston, *Missionary Travels*, 94–97, 241, 573, 612.

77. Ibid., 241.

78. Haggard, 49–50. Anne McClintock argues the journey in the novel is a journey through the ideological space of Africa. See McClintock, 244.

79. Du Chaillu, 182.

80. Ibid., 180.

81. Owen Fletcher, *The Bonds of Africa: Impressions of Travel and Sport from Cape Town to Cairo, 1902–1912* (London: J. Long, 1913), 242.

82. Oswald, 128.

83. Kirkland, 163.

84. Ibid.

85. Thornhill, ix.

86. Tucker.

87. Purvis.

88. Ibid., 146.

89. K.C. Willet, "Trypanosomiasis Research at Tinde," *Tanganyika Notes and Records* 34(1953), 33–34.

90. McKelvey, 207–238.

91. Vaughan, 158, 175.

92. Winston Churchill, *My African Journey* (London: Hodder, 1908).

93. Ibid.

94. Ibid., 99–102.

95. Ibid., 94–103.

96. J. Speke, 262.

97. David William Cohen, "Peoples and States of the Great Lakes Region," in J. F. Ade Ajayi, ed., *General History of Africa*, vol. 6 (London, 1989), 270–293.

98. M. S. M. Kiwanuka, *A History of Buganda* (New York, 1972), 195; Ray, 132.

99. Stanley, 230.

100. Kiwanuka, 140–143.

101. Ashe, 161.

102. Cunningham, 77–78; Hartwig, 378.

103. H. B. Thomas and Robert Scott, *Uganda* (London, 1935), 31–32; Ashe, 161.

104. Twaddle, 45–47.

105. Roscoe, 271–345.

106. Ray, 132.

107. Kimwanuka, 138; Stanley, 207.

108. Kimwanuka, 195.

109. Ibid., 138; Stanley, 207.

110. Twaddle, 88–91.

111. L. A. Fallers, *Bantu Bureaucracy* (Chicago, 1965), 38, 42, 145; Twaddle, 221–224.

112. John Beattie, *Bunyoro: An African Kingdom*, (New York, 1960), 19–22.

113. Cohen, "Natur und Kampf," 10–23.

114. Roscoe, 17.

115. Busoga Protectorate Agent Alexander Boyle, 1906, quoted in Twaddle, 223; Fallers, 146.

116. Fallers, 309.

117. Cohen, "Natur und Kampf," 15–18.

118. Soff, "A History of Sleeping Sickness," 3–13.

119. Bell, 114. Regents received 400 pounds annually, and Saza chiefs 200 pounds annually. The Uganda Agreement is reprinted in D. A. Low, *The Mind of Buganda* (London, 1971), 32–36.

120. A. Richards, *Subsistence to Commercial Farming*, 67–68.

121. Holger Bernt Hansen, *Mission, Church, and State in a Colonial Setting: Uganda, 1890–1925* (New York, 1984), 106–107.

122. R. Van Zwanberg, *An Economic History of Kenya and Uganda* (London, 1975); W. Elkan, *The Economic Development of Uganda* (London, 1961); J. Jorgensen, *Uganda A Modern History* (New York, 1981).

123. Robert W. July, *A History of the African People* (New York, 1980), 468.

124. David E. Apter, *The Political Economy in Uganda* (Princeton, 1967), 49.

125. Ibid., 226–233, 256–261.

126. Ibid., 310–326.

127. Portal, 182.

128. A. Richards, *Changing Structure*, 20.

129. A. Richards, *Subsistence to Commercial Farming*, 60.

130. Hansen, 92.

131. Tucker, 287.

132. Fallers, 50, 127, 136; Cohen, *The Historical Tradition of Busoga*, 16–19.

133. Twaddle, 89–90; Twaddle argues Sesse canoe crews were Bugandan slaves, but considering the political relationship between the kingdom and the islands, they probably were tributary forced labor as opposed to the war and slave captives from Busoga and Buvuma. See "The Ending of Slavery in Buganda," in Suzanne Meirs and Richard Roberts, eds., *The End of Slavery in Africa* (Madison, 1988), 125–126.

134. Roscoe, 310–311.

CHAPTER 3

Depopulations and Safe Corridors in Colonial Uganda, 1906–1920

Barring one small affray in one village in which three people were wounded, there has not been the slightest conflict with people.
Governor Hesketh Bell, 1907[1]

At Wambeti we used to land to trade, but suddenly it was deserted. We didn't know where to go to trade, and whether the whites would confiscate our canoes.
Samuel Kinbya[2]

In 1906 colonial administrators began declaring certain areas as epidemic or potentially epidemic environments and outlawing human occupation for that reason. For purposes of surveillance, communication, and commerce, they ordered that African labor should keep a limited number of authorized roads and landings within official infected areas clear of brush to allow people on business deemed essential to the political and economic well-being of the region to move safely through otherwise depopulated territory. This chapter examines the relationship between officially designated infected areas and fly-free corridors, with particular focus on the Lake Victoria Infected Area, in terms of the construction of new spatial arrangements in Uganda and in terms of the political and economic considerations that influenced sleeping sickness control.

By 1910 the colonial administration had declared six infected areas in Uganda, most on the geopolitical margins of the protectorate (see figure 3.1). Africans affected by depopulations did not understand sleeping sickness control policy as disease control, or did not understand sleeping sickness control policy as merely disease control. The historic experience of Ganda fishers and farmers relocating within the Buganda kingdom was in accordance with the state reallotment of elite landholdings. On the other hand, non-Ganda who were removed from infected areas as a result of the cooperation between British and Ganda authorities viewed sleeping sickness control within the context of Buganda imperial expansion. The geographic locations of most depopulated areas permitted the consolidation of Buganda state power over people historically opposed to the extension of Buganda political hegemony.

The Lake Victoria Infected Area was the first, and reportedly most virulent, infected sleeping sickness area in Uganda. The lakeshore of Busoga to the east of the Nile River was the focus of the turn-of-the-century epidemic. Missionaries and colonial scientists reported cases in other designated infected areas, for example in the Bunyoro and Lake Albert Areas, but these numbers were small compared to the dramatic death rate along Lake Victoria. Other than the Lake Victoria Infected Area, the colonial state depopulated the other areas because of tsetse infestation and risk of epidemic.

The Lake Victoria Area was a two-mile-wide strip running the entire length of southern Uganda, including all of the Lake Victoria islands designated as part of Uganda in the 1900 Uganda Agreement. Sleeping sickness control plans for this infected area relocated people from southern Buganda, southern Busoga, the Sesse Islands, and the Buvuma Islands. The colonial state began forcing people to leave the mainland fly zone in late 1906 and to vacate the islands beginning in 1908. The state reopened this infected area for settlement in a piecemeal fashion—starting with parts of the mainland as early as 1910 and extending to the islands after 1912. By 1920 colonial health officials decided the sleeping sickness emergency was over and in accordance with this decision in 1924 they officially reopened most infected areas for resettlement. Some 15 years later, sleeping sickness officials revised this decision, once more depopulating a more limited area of southern Busoga, including some lake islands. This second depopulation was maintained from 1941 through the 1960s and 1970s when the national state took over the task. Despite the limited nature and minimal enforcement of depopulation policies between 1941 and 1962, the colonial state vigorously applied components of the sleeping sickness control regulations whenever officials reported cases of sleeping sickness or dangerous degrees of tsetse fly infestation.[3] Significantly, neither the British nor the post-1962 Uganda national state ever reopened all of the Lake Victoria mainland shore and islands for settlement and unregulated fishing. The colonial state permanently confiscated parts of infected areas after both depopulations by recategorizing them as crown lands, forest reserves, and game sanctuaries.

Buganda internal politics informed the enactment of sleeping sickness policies through 1920. Colonial and Ganda leadership came to agree upon many depopulation orders; such orders percolated down through various African political hierarchies until finally reaching the village level. The ways that local

Figure 3.1
Uganda Official Infected Areas, 1912

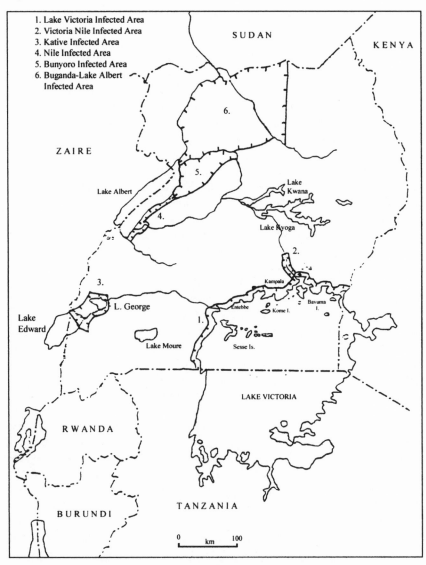

1. Lake Victoria Infected Area
2. Victoria Nile Infected Area
3. Kative Infected Area
4. Nile Infected Area
5. Bunyoro Infected Area
6. Buganda-Lake Albert
   Infected Area

SUDAN

KENYA

ZAIRE

6.

5.

Lake Albert

Lake
Kwana

4.

Lake Kyoga

2.

Kampala

3.

L. George

Bavuma
I.

Entebbe

Kome I.

Lake
Edward

1.

Lake Moure

Sesse Is.

LAKE VICTORIA

RWANDA

BURUNDI

TANZANIA

0   km   100

Based on a map, UNA, 1912.

African leaders, farmers, and fishers responded to depopulation schemes—and to the state's (colonial and African) authority and ability to enforce its decisions—altered British views of Uganda, tropical environments, and Africans as actors within these environments.

STRATEGIES OF DEPOPULATION

Depopulation as a solution to sleeping sickness reveals several distinct images the British held of Uganda and betrays the relationship between science and colonization which developed in the context of informal colonial rule and the Uganda Agreement. The mission of disease intervention brought together an array of groups who then jockeyed amongst themselves for positions within an emerging colonial bureaucratic system. Colonial administrators found it necessary to weigh the issue of expense and their desire to construct profitable colonial economies against the complications engendered by political alliances struck with African elite and with local farmers and fishers. Furthermore, British administrators had to keep in mind the many (conflicting at this time) obligations involved in the civilizing mission during a period of perceived epidemic emergency.

British colonial officials held conflicting interests. In 1906 the district commissioner of Busoga and the principle medical officer of Uganda (A. D. P. Hodges) disagreed about strategies of tsetse control. The district commissioner argued, using the profit motive, to have Africans hand-catch tsetse: "We might begin by offering a shell apiece. At that rate an expenditure of 20 pounds should ensure the destruction of 15,000 flies. As soon as the flies become scarcer through collection, the price will have to be raised, and if by offering sufficient rewards for their capture we can ensure their almost complete extermination in this stricken country, 20,000 pounds would not be too high a price to pay!"[4] His primary concern lay with the financial cost of ending an epidemic in the region. A sleeping-sickness epidemic was threatening the availability of Soga labor before it could be put to British advantage. In the commissioner's view, a harmonious administrative and ideological solution to the problem would be to attach a profit motive to the collection of tsetse flies; such a plan might put an end to fly infestations and serve to organize African labor as well. To the contrary, Dr. Hodges suggested that the control of sleeping sickness in Uganda lay beyond the power of economic incentives and stressed the need for education and ongoing scientific research and intervention.[5]

The new governor of Uganda, Hesketh Bell, outlined a depopulation plan for the Lake Victoria shore in late 1906 but was unable to get official approval from London because of disagreement between scientists and administrators. For the previous six years, reports from missionaries, colonial scientists, officials, and travelers and reports from local African elite had been clearly identifying the epidemic area and the high death toll. Colonial scientists had made the link between sleeping sickness and tsetse three years prior. Bell, frustrated that the colonial office in London was not responding to his requests to depopulate epidemic areas, independently initiated his plans in late 1906. He finally received the approval of the colonial office in late 1907 after traveling to London to present the office with the depopulation of the lakeshore as, in his own words, a "fait accompli."[6]

Colonial administrators in England were concerned that forced depopulations in Uganda would create tensions over land tenure and the availability of unoccupied fertile land and that socioeconomic disruptions might incite popular resistance.[7] According to Bell, primary opposition to his plan from the colonial office came from Patrick Manson, who was discussed in the previous chapter. Bell wrote that Manson initially opposed ideas for forced depopulations, arguing they would lead to a "serious native war" over of the question of land.[8] In Uganda the depopulation idea prevailed in response to the perception of the sleeping sickness epidemic as a drastic and immediate threat to people's lives. This included concerns about the population as a productive workforce and African health as an indicator of colonial legitimacy. The implementation of depopulations in Uganda reinforced colonial notions that African labor could be moved around and that people were not particularly connected to specific lands. An assumption behind sleeping sickness depopulations in Uganda was that because of environmental fertility and the effectiveness of centralized state control, farmers could reestablish the same production systems wherever they ended up.

Bell collaborated with Hodges, who was based in Jinja just east of the mouth of the Victoria Nile, in formulating the specifics of the first emergency intervention. Hodges had begun to experiment with tsetse-control schemes to protect Entebbe in 1904, and both men were familiar with ongoing Royal Society research.[9] Sleeping sickness ordinances in 1907 ordered the depopulation of all land from the Lake Victoria shore two miles inland, including the lake islands. The plan reflected early scientific research on sleeping sickness and tsetse and pointed future research in specific directions, such as where tsetse flourished, how long infected tsetse fly remained infected, and how far tsetse could travel. The counting and mapping of tsetse and disease deaths marked the emergence of new field methods for epidemiology and entomology. Sleeping sickness scientists employed African men as "fly boys" to collect tsetse, both dead and alive, from specific locations. Colonial sleeping sickness scientists then noted how many tsetse were caught in different places in what time period by how many fly boys to begin to assess preferred tsetse habitats, cycles of activity, trypanosome infection rates, and movements.[10] The two-mile line along Lake Victoria was set back from what research and reports showed as the center of disease deaths and tsetse closer to the lake in order to create a buffer zone between occupied lands and diseased environments.

But the two-mile line also reflected politics of land alienation. Massive state alienation of productive land conflicted with colonial ideas of Ganda productivity and informal rule through the Buganda state. The British struggled to reconcile forced depopulations with the idea of civilized governance, the Uganda Agreement, and any expectations of African cooperation.[11] Unlike its rationale of permanent alienation of land for white settlers as allowing more rational and efficient agricultural production, the colonial state justified sleeping sickness depopulations scientifically as temporary emergency health measures. The colonial state would hold the lands in public trust until scientists judged them safe for reoccupation. This policy gave power to colonial scientists. It necessitated continuous research in infected areas to legitimize ongoing, but supposedly temporary, depopulation.

The idea of Africans' responsibility for the spread of sleeping sickness helped the colonial state justify enforcing mass population removals. The scientific idea behind depopulations was to segregate people temporarily from unhealthy environments. Theoretically, if denied the human reservoir of trypanosomes, fly populations would eventually become infection free. But scientists were in the process of determining that tsetse flies received trypanosomes from biting infected bodies, that is, they merely carried the infection to their next food source. Humans, in effect, could only receive the disease from other infected humans, flies being a vector of transmission as opposed to the source of disease. Scientists did not yet recognize that wildlife were a reservoir for human trypanosomiasis as well. This substantiated a mythology that nature was not inherently disordered and could purify itself if given enough time.

Thus, the scientific explanation of sleeping sickness shared blame between flies and Africans. It was Africans who carried within them the kernels of disease, being both victims and agents of its spread. In colonial eyes, local Africans became responsible for the disorder of their environment that allowed fly infestation by living in unhealthy space and therefore being disordered themselves. The Entebbe Township Ordinance of 1906 allowed the inspection of canoes and people at lake landings or offshore. If a health inspector found a tsetse fly on board, "the owner and crew shall be deemed to have committed an offense and shall be liable for punishment as upon a breech of these rules unless they shall prove that due care and diligence was used." The fine was 100 rupees or up to one month imprisonment, or both.[12] A convenience of scientific knowledge was that because colonial officials understood it to be by definition objective, scientifically determined transgressions became indefensible. Scientific justifications for depopulations, therefore, transcended all moral and political objections to the policy.

That depopulations were to be temporary was important to securing African state and local cooperation. According to the mechanisms of informal British power in Uganda, depopulations could only occur with the cooperation of African leaders ordering people to move, and British officials believed land alienation was a central Ganda-elite concern. The three regents of the young Kabaka Daudi Chwa, regional Saza chiefs, and other Ganda notables on the National Council were concerned about the status of infected areas as a category of landholdings and about the duration of closings.[13] Chief Kweba of the Sesses and Chief Mbubi of Buvuma asked in 1909, "How long shall it be before we go back to our country, is it certain that when the Sleeping Sickness has come to an end we shall return to the islands?"[14]

The control of land had been a central issue in the 1900 Uganda Agreement. The sleeping sickness control plan tested British informal rule enacted through the Uganda Agreement. Local Africans perceived the depopulation of infected areas, in part, as a new twist on British land accumulation. In 1921, when the colonial government claimed some depopulated sleeping sickness lands on the Sesse Islands as crown lands, Kabaka Daudi Chwa pondered, "One might think that perhaps there was another reason why the people were removed from the Sesse Islands."[15] Ganda elite weighed this suspicion against the advantages of *mailo* holdings, salaries, and the British support of Ganda political positions that came with cooperation.

The political issue of how long infected areas would be closed paralleled the scientific process of determining how long trypanosomes lived in tsetse flies. These experiments justified, and were justified by, the vector separation theory. Through 1908 colonial scientists estimated that a 48-hour human/fly vector separation was enough to render fly populations infection free.[16] Then in 1910 David Bruce, an army doctor and chair of the second Royal Society commission who ran over 30 experiments on the duration of trypanosome infestation in tsetse in Uganda, revised the 48-hour estimate: "It has been found by experiment that fly can retain its infectivity up to 80 days. It is probable that after a fly has become infected it will harbour the trypanosomes for the rest of its life; but what the duration of this is, under natural conditions, is unknown."[17] Bruce advocated that the Buvuma be given assurances that they would be allowed to return to their island after three years. The acting British governor, Stanley Tomkins, decided that because of the uncertainty of the duration of infection he would make no such guarantee.[18] The inability of colonial science to resolve definitively the time frame of environmental self-purification left ambiguous the political commitment to resettlement.

As discussed in chapter 2, the geopolitical locations of infected areas hint at other strategic reasons for Ganda elite cooperation with sleeping sickness control measures. The declaration of infected areas consolidated Ganda power over the margins. All infected areas were on the borders of Ganda political authority. The Bunyoro and Buganda Infected Areas declared in 1909 depopulated the northern part of what was left of Bunyoro under the authority of British and Ganda officials. The Uganda Agreement made Buvuma a reluctant district of Buganda, and the depopulation of Buvuma as "infected" increased Ganda power over the island group. The Victoria Nile sleeping sickness area followed the border between Buganda and Busoga. The Bunyoro Infected Area, Buganda (Lake Albert) Infected Area, and the islands in the

Lake Victoria Infected Area were in centers of historic political resistance to Ganda hegemony.

The depopulation of Buvuma, the Sesse Islands, the Busoga coast, and large parts of Bunyoro, as well as the consolidation of populations closer to the Buganda core, and the policing of these areas by Ganda officials working under the auspices of the colonial state in the name of health, were to Ganda state advantage. The Kabaka's objection to crown lands on the Sesse Islands was not in defense of islanders' land rights but because the British were allowing only former residents to repopulate the Sesses. Thus the British were denying Ganda settlement of the islands.[19] On the northeastern side of the lake, Ganda officials used sleeping sickness regulations in 1910 to try to depopulate Kenyan islands as part of the Lake Victoria Infected Area, thereby extending Ganda territorial claims.[20]

Expedition reports by Royal Society Sleeping Sickness Commissions reflect scientific attention directed outward to the margins of Buganda. Early sleeping sickness tours in 1904 and 1905 explored the strategically important Nile Valley. During E. D. W. Greig's sleeping sickness tour of Lake Albert and the Nile Valley, he linked up with a gunboat and a British colonial medical officer from Egypt, Dr. Sheffield, "sent by the Egyptian Government to co-operate with me to investigate the banks of the Nile."[21] Cooperation here between Egypt, the British colonial state in Uganda, and the Ganda state shows how sleeping sickness control joined together different imperial agendas. Colonial explorer-scientists operated on the outskirts of known territory. The colonial periphery of the Buganda empire became the periphery of the British colonial state. British officials were doing disease surveys at newly established government posts in Buvuma, Busoga, Toro, Bunyoro, and the Ruwenzori mountains.[22] Colonial scientific expeditions to discover and declare areas of sleeping sickness followed the routes of past British military expeditions which had, in turn, followed the routes of Ganda military expeditions.

MAKING PEOPLE MOVE

The Department of Health and Hygiene administered sleeping sickness control. British sleeping sickness officers from that department designated homesteads and villages as legal or illegal. In November 1906 the colonial government gave chiefs administering lands on the Lake Victoria shore in Buganda and Busoga three months to move people inland. Officials then counted huts in infected areas and disseminated evacuation orders. Officials organized local labor to erect road and path barriers.[23] Some family members went ahead to prepare fields and begin building new homes, while others gathered as much food as could be harvested and transported before eviction. Households packed what they could transport by foot and moved in one or more primary trips.[24] For a short time after the March deadline, people were allowed to return to former homesteads to harvest food as it became ripe.[25]

Beginning in March, police parties burnt abandoned homes and *shambas* to deter illegal returns.[26]

Sleeping sickness officials reported depopulations went smoothly and successfully on the mainland. They stressed that chiefs were helpful in evacuation and the people responsive. Governor Bell wrote in June 1907 that "barring one small affray in one village in which three people were wounded, there has not been the slightest conflict with people."[27] His explanation of popular acquiescence was that "lower classes have always been so thoroughly under the control of their chiefs that the idea of resistance to the wishes of the government in this matter doubtless never entered into their minds."[28] By promoting this image of Ganda cooperation, Bell assuaged concerns in Britain about his sleeping sickness policies. He also affirmed the British vision of the Buganda state as effective, efficient, and legitimate.

Local farmers' and fishers' oral accounts and local colonial accounts reflect more differentiated regional and personal responses. Histories of land tenure in the various states and regions conditioned African responses and understandings of depopulations. Sleeping sickness policies were least contested in mainland Buganda. Ganda farmers were familiar with the idea of politically determined evictions and relocations. Coming soon after the political, socio-economic, and environmental disruptions of the late nineteenth century and the land restructuring of the Uganda Agreement, the sleeping sickness forced relocations were not unusual for Ganda farmers.

The colonial government tried to expedite the process to minimize any risk of popular resistance. The British paid five shillings in compensation to each refugee household that applied for restitution for destroyed homes and fields and suspended its taxes for one to two years.[29] After March 1911 the colonial administration did not consider any further compensation cases, although over 1,000 were pending. The administration considered relocations made that late too delinquent to merit compensation.[30] In 1906 the government published "Explanatory Address on Sleeping Sickness to the Natives of the Uganda Protectorate." This was 13 pages of explanations, directives, and pleas by Dr. Hodges about the necessity of sleeping sickness regulations and the importance of keeping homesteads and roads well cleared of bush. The document was published in English and Kiganda but not translated into Lusoga or Lunyoro, emphasizing the exclusionary nature of the English-Ganda relationship.[31]

Responses in Busoga, Buvuma, and the Sesse Islands were less acquiescent. Soga oral sources emphasized the threat of imprisonment (2 months hard labor in 1908 increased to 12 months in 1910) and the idea that homes would be burned whether inhabited or not.[32] Some hid the sick from sleeping sickness authorities hoping this would save them from eviction. Oral sources maintained many families would have preferred to risk staying on their lands. The colonial administration mandated fines and prison sentences for people caught in closed areas without permits. Sleeping sickness officers conducted boat and land patrols to confiscate or destroy boats, possessions, and gardens found in infected areas, and to apprehend anyone in the areas after March 1, 1909. Chiefs were assigned responsibility over borders of the infected areas and could be fined if colonial officers discovered people had trespassed into infected areas across their borders.[33] Soga emphasized these were coerced removals.[34]

Sleeping sickness officials extended depopulation policy to the Lake Victoria islands from 1909 to 1911, and islander resistance was overt. The people of Lake Victoria during the eighteenth and nineteenth centuries were both excluded from mainland state power and better able to maintain independence from it. The lake environment and resources, as well as canoe transportation, afforded lake people mobility and adaptability, allowing them the option of withdrawal from state encroachment but also making them valuable (as naval power) to the state. Island political structures were thus more resistant to depopulation orders, and the people more elusive and suspicious of land alienation by a Ganda-British alliance.

Buvuma and Sesse islanders placed sleeping sickness depopulations in the context of their historic experiences with Buganda—military invasions, slave raids, and demands for tribute. In 1910 an armed group of Ganda, falsely claiming to represent the sleeping sickness authorities, murdered people and seized property and slaves on several Buvuma islands.[35] Islanders thus met official Ganda sleeping sickness guards and police with suspicion and hostility. Two Ganda sleeping sickness guards sent to remove people from Buvuma Island in 1909 estimated thousands of "illegal" inhabitants, led by uncooperative chiefs, refused to leave. The guards withdrew.[36]

Beginning in 1908 colonial disease control attempted a process of island consolidation. Health regulations ordered the populations of 33 lake islands to consolidate on 13 islands.[37] Then in April 1909 the colonial administration gazetted all lake islands closed and gave islanders two months to leave. Sesse islanders were to move to the Buganda Buddu mainland directly to their west. Buvuma residents, officially subjects of Buganda since the Uganda Agreement, were to relocate to Kyagwe between Kampala and Jinja. Islanders responded to evacuation orders with negotiations, overt resistance, and desertion. By July sleeping sickness officials recorded the relocation of 2,300 Sesse islanders out of an estimated total 12,000 and 34 of an estimated 11,000 total Buvuma.[38]

The responses of local people to sleeping sickness control ordinances also differed according to where the state intended to move people. The Buganda state benefited from the consolidation of marginal populations into the Buganda core. Organized sleeping sickness fleets moved islanders to the mainland. Many Buvuma moved independently to Busoga instead of being relocated in Buganda. Mainland and island elite were concerned about the loss of power and people. The two-mile line did not place any Ganda province completely within the infected area, and most displaced mainland farmers and fishers resettled close to former lands, usually within the same province. Ganda and Soga chiefs, then, lost territory but not that many clientele.

Island elite lost both land and people. Among the questions Chief Kweba of the Sesses and Chief Mbubi of Buvuma asked in 1909 during negotiations with sleeping sickness authorities were whether they would continue to draw their pay and whether their people would be settled on unproductive mainland land: "We hear that we shall be free from the payment of taxes for 2 years. The time should be more, 3 years. Where shall such people get food when they live on waste land? Shall we the saza chiefs continue drawing our pay?"[39] The colonial governor rejected the three-year deadline, and payment of chiefs' salaries was to be contingent on successful depopulation efforts. After continued resistance, in 1911 the British administration assured island chiefs political independence on the mainland: "For political reasons, keep relocated Sesse and Buvuma people as units, preserving their identity, and not merging with the Ganda race, reporting to their own chiefs. All are to pay taxes through the DC Kampala."[40] In theory this meant the formation of distinct new villages, but such villages were never formed, and many island elite became common farmers on the mainland.[41] But with reluctant and inconsistent support by elite and local missionaries for the disease-control orders, Buvuma and Sesse islanders began to relocate.

Some island residents refused and retreated with canoes and belongings to smaller islands, into papyrus swamps and island hills. Health officials responded with force. Chief Mbubi and armed police pursued resistors in the forests of Buvuma Island, and the chief was wounded in a subsequent skirmish. The police killed several resistors, and a group of 200 Buvuma, mostly women and children, surrendered the next day.[42] When people fled sleeping sickness officials, police destroyed the homes, crops, boats, and possessions they had left behind. People were threatened with fines and imprisonment. By November 1909, 11,000 Buvuma were resettled on the mainland, but by May 1910 fishers and farmers illegally inhabited the island again. The Bavuma argued they were dying on the mainland anyway. A second Ganda-British expedition in October burned *shambas* and recaptured 3,000 squatters settled farther inland.[43]

Health officials did not have the resources to police all the islands. Most colonial scientists left Uganda during World War I, and from 1913 through 1918 there were few sleeping sickness area inspections.[44] While colonial officers depopulated the more visible and accessible population centers on larger islands such as Sigulu, Buvuma, and Bugala by 1911, the British were aware that illegal occupants remained throughout the islands.

The British perceived islanders as most likely to be infected and most likely to be transporting trypanosome and flies along with cargoes of fish and other trade goods between settled areas. Health officials considered fishers particularly dangerous because their movements were difficult to regulate. Colonialists' primary experience with lake people was as they appeared at landings to unload fish, register, buy supplies, and then disappear again onto the lake.

After an effort at depopulating islands and controlling movement, sleeping sickness regulations legally cut off the islands from the mainland. Sleeping sickness ordinances made fishing within two miles of the shore illegal and the sale or possession of lake fish an offense.[45] Because British officials found mainland environments easier to order, and relatively easily moved mainland farmers to new farmlands, they prioritized disease control on the mainland. Health officials categorized islanders as a threat to be countered, as opposed to a people to be saved. During initial Sesse depopulations, medical officers gave immigrants blood tests as they landed on the mainland and returned the sick to the islands to die. This practice contradicted the scientific plan of vector isolation, the humanitarianism of colonial medicine, and the politics of depopulation. Africans and colonial officials objected, and the policy was ended.[46]

ORDERED ACCESS

While colonial scientists determined the form and extent of depopulated areas, the policy of limited strategic clearings which allowed controlled human access in the infected areas reflected other colonial interests. Scientists had shown that tsetse fly avoided hot, open spaces. Therefore, for reasons of economics, political control, and access to basic resources, local labor was to keep certain landings and roads fly free by bush and papyrus clearing and tree thinning. Legal clearings included major roads and river fords in the northern infected areas, numerous Lake Victoria landings, and connecting roads in the Lake Victoria Infected Area.

Scientists and health officials were not involved in deciding where access would be allowed, but they did conceive the form for these ordered spaces. The colonial government printer published sleeping sickness officer Dr. Hodges's original 1907 clearing-scheme drawings in revised form in a 1911 pamphlet. Sleeping sickness control plans mandated that African labor would clear essential ports and ferry landings 200 yards deep and one-half mile in either direction. Hodges's general-lakeshore-clearing plan began on the waterfront with a 20-yard, completely cleared, "inner belt" and then extended back in three gradually increasing belt widths: from 30, to 50, to 100 yards (see figure 3.2). There was a certain flexibility within the space in terms of the number of trees allowed.[47] Belt 2 could contain up to 5 trees per acre lopped to 15 feet from the ground. Belt 3 was to be lopped "to 10 feet from the ground, and not more than 15 trees per acre," and belt 4 could have up to 30 trees per acre with no lopping required. Here was the vision of a gradually flowing transition from open land to bush, from light to shadow, and from health to disease. It was a visual acknowledgment that colonial order must coexist with environmental chaos, but a chaos defined and circumscribed.

But the logic of this lakeshore plan was to separate two essential parts of fly habitat—water and shade—and thus eventually render both environments sleeping sickness free. The gradual thinning out of trees closer to the lake was meant to make the shore increasingly unattractive to flies. Hodges's attention to tree density had an economic, as well as an esthetic, component: "But a certain number of timber trees can always be spared if so desired, and it will be rarely that any particular tree can not be preserved with safety." Hodges's plan combined the esthetic interests of the botanical gardener with colonial economic concerns about the clearing of hardwoods and the rubber vines they carried.

Diagrams of control plans for human access at landings, fords, and ferries were triangular with a straight central road maximizing walking distance through the clearing from bush to beach to leave flies behind (see figure 3.3). Hodges showed how to apply his vision to irregular shorelines, and how to take water currents into account at river ferries and fords. He based the plans on geometric precision and the control of human and fly movement. All people (if they kept to the legal path) were to travel 300 yards through shade-free, fly-free cleared land from the lake to the forest, or from the forest to the lake. The area within a triangle formed by a 600-yard lakeshore base (300 yards on each side of the road head at figure 3.3, point C) and a 300-yard height, to where the road proceeded into the forest was to be cleared. People could stay within the cleared space except for 100-yard-wide quadrangles on the far sides that were to be "railed off and should be taboo." The diagram-defined forest area for flies where people were prohibited, cleared space for people that flies would supposedly avoid, and cleared spaces (where forest and water came closest together) denied to people as well.

Hodges overlaid human and tsetse behaviors on an abstracted, esthetic sense of environmental order related to straight lines and neat angles. A further adjustment in the 1911 landings diagram allowed for a few shade trees, "but no bush, scrub or long grass," in the central area near the access path. He had reports that fishers, traders, and travelers at clearings were not keeping on the central path away from flies, as women fetching water preferred to walk and rest in the shade, and canoe crews tended to off-load in cooler clearing edges. Hodges revised his response to Uganda behavior. He made allowances for shade but in the center of ordered space: "If there are no suitable trees, shelters, preferably open sheds at least six feet high at the eaves, may be erected. In the absence of shade natives cannot be prevented from eating, sleeping, etc., in the surrounding jungle. It will be best, where there is considerable traffic, to provide some sort of latrine accommodation in cleared area."[48] Hodges's revision joined plant, fly, and human "physics" with acknowledgments of the limits of colonial power—that only so much bush could be cleared—and acknowledgment of how people were acting at landings.

Figure 3.2
Diagram of Cleared Beach, Uganda

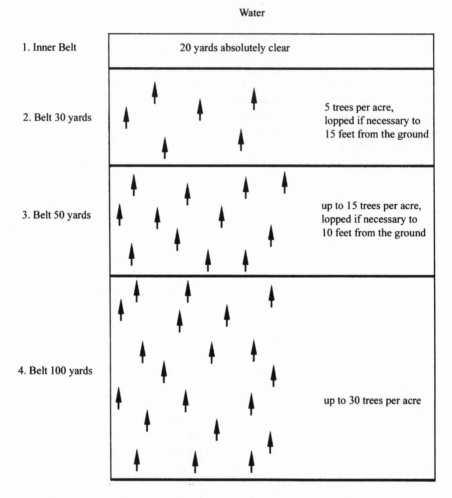

Water

1. Inner Belt   20 yards absolutely clear

2. Belt 30 yards   5 trees per acre,
lopped if necessary to
15 feet from the ground

3. Belt 50 yards   up to 15 trees per acre,
lopped if necessary to
10 feet from the ground

4. Belt 100 yards   up to 30 trees per acre

Based on a drawing in A. D. P. Hodges, *Sleeping Sickness Clearning Scheme* (Entebbe, 1911).

In the practical context of narrow, cleared strips passing through forbidden (depopulated) infected areas, the selection and maintenance of official clearings caused confusion for Africans and conflict between colonial interest groups. The primary purpose of the cleared landings was to maintain essential communication and commerce on the lake. But Buganda state officials were concerned about the disruption of internal trade and also about the hypocrisy of special consideration given to white concessionaires. For instance, after

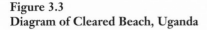

Figure 3.3
Diagram of Cleared Beach, Uganda

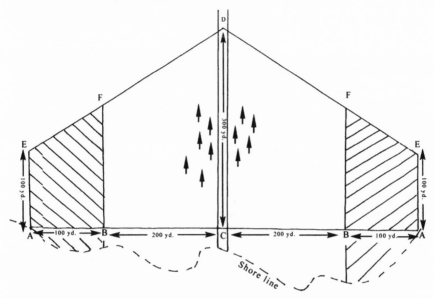

Based on a drawing from A. D. P. Hodges, *Sleeping Sickness Scheme* (Entebbe, 1911).

Ganda officials had ordered workers for L. Campbell, a white concessionaire, out of the Nasagasa Forest in the Lake Victoria sleeping sickness area, he received special permission for his workers to continue gathering rubber, as long as he housed them outside the infected area.[49]

The 1908 Sleeping Sickness Ordinance declared 17 mainland, 17 Sesse, and 10 Buvuma landings and the connecting roads open (cleared) for use.[50] But the colonial administration continuously revised these locations as it balanced medical concerns with economic and military needs for efficient lake access. The question of the transportation of cattle between Bukakata and Bugala Island, for example, prompted a debate in 1908 about the tension between the health risks of cattle, human, and fly movement and the economic necessity of such transport. Colonial officers carried on a similar discussion about how vital subsistence-food imports from the mainland were to certain Buvuma islands yet to be declared closed.[51] The course of such debates changed which mainland landings received clearing attention.

Sleeping sickness control clearing initiated a long colonial process of experimentation with the most efficient and cost-effective uses of labor and technology. Maintaining cleared landings counterposed medical and fiscal interests. Official clearing teams of African labor, equipped and supervised by sleeping sickness authorities, implemented Hodges's plan. To maintain landings, however, sleeping sickness officers had to organize local labor on a regular basis. Colonial administrators sought to minimize labor party movements over the two-mile barrier, so they tried to maintain a permanent population at landings capable of carrying out necessary clearing. They faced a conundrum: too many people increased the health risks of epidemic, while too few people couldn't do the necessary clearing thus increasing the health risk of flies. The Uganda Protectorate Annual Medical and Sanitary Report of 1938 warned, "A neglected clearing is more dangerous than the original forest."[52] In 1908 sleeping sickness officials closed the gazetted landing at Buira and burned all structures because there were not enough regular inhabitants to keep it clear.[53] Colonial health authorities denied a local petition to reopen the Wairaka landing in 1930 because only 25 people wished to return, and this was deemed not enough to do the necessary clearing work.[54]

Lake people were also extremely mobile, moving legally and illegally with changing market opportunities, so it proved difficult to enforce the colonial sense of order dependent on stable habitation. Health regulations created conditions that increased illegal movement. Sleeping sickness officials regularly checked work parties and landing populations for trypanosomes. Africans in infected areas had to carry up-to-date medical permits at all times. Colonial scientists used these groups for drug experiments.[55]

Sleeping sickness authorities monitored landing populations and maintenance and recommended closures and openings to the governor. The process of closing and opening landings involved counting people and flies, clearing people and vegetation, organizing and medically testing labor, and keeping local people in the middle of roads in plain sight. Health issues combined with shifting perceptions of which landings were most strategically vital to the colonial mandate to create numerous changes in the list of legal landings. On January 1, 1909, the *Uganda Gazette* published a new list of official closures and openings and updated this list monthly. Sleeping sickness authorities closed Bugoma on January 30 and opened Jiba on July 17. They opened Kisubi and Katotis on August 4 and closed Banga, Kibanga, Nansangazi, and Kasirye on October 30.[56] Farmers, fishers, and traders found this process difficult to understand and abide by and, thereby, couldn't help landing "illegally" and using closed lands: "At Wambeti we used to land to trade, but suddenly it was deserted. We didn't know where to go to trade, and if the whites would confiscate our canoes."[57]

In the construction of depopulated infected areas and gazetted legal roads and landings through these areas, and in the policing of legal and illegal spaces, colonial scientists and health officials developed a complicated system of monitoring and controlling people and environments. The two-part system of sleeping sickness control in Uganda created self-perpetuating, scientific problems to solve. Depopulated areas turned to forest, making colonial policing more difficult. Without constant maintenance, strategic gazetted clearings quickly became overgrown as well. From a colonial perspective, broader colonial goals, scientific knowledge and methods, and environmental and demographic conditions changed over time, necessitating a process of landing openings and closings. From a local African perspective, the colonial logic of sleeping sickness control was illusive. The British admired Ganda and Soga agricultural production, then forced valuable lands to be abandoned. Forests consequently expanded, and the British were exasperated at African failures to clear them back properly at certain places and in certain shapes.

EMPTIED LANDS

For both the mainland and islands, Ugandan oral sources and colonial sources agree that the depopulation of infected areas was generally effective in terms of removing and then barring permanent settlement. For the most part in closed areas, underbrush and forest reclaimed homesteads and banana plantations, and signs of long-term human habitation disappeared. Police and research teams observed forest quickly filling in homesteads and fields. A sleeping sickness inspector wrote after touring the depopulated Busoga lakeshore, "Vines and thorned underbrush have quickly grown over former plantations and vegetable gardens. The forest expands very quickly. It is eerie to feel as if no one has been here for hundreds of years. It will soon be difficult to distinguish former fields and villages."[58] Here was the theoretical recreation of Africa as nature, left to bring itself to scientifically determined order through the removal of human inhabitants.

The Lake Victoria islands took on a particular meaning for colonial science. Colonial scientists took advantage of emptied islands as isolated, self-contained research and testing grounds. Research conclusions were based on island trypanosome, fly, and animal populations being isolated from human contact and uncontaminated by any new tsetse or trypanosomes Africans might transport. Scientific expeditions regularly toured the islands starting in 1910 as Africans left. From 1910 to 1914 research teams, with crews of Ganda workers, established camps on Damba, Bugalla, Kome, and Lwagi Islands in the Buvuma and Sesse groups. The research teams conducted experiments on the duration of trypanosome infection, habitat, and life span of tsetse. For experiments on animals hosts, scientists became particularly interested in isolated populations of situtunga antelope found on the islands.[59] In 1926 the state permanently alienated Damba Island as a scientific reserve to protect antelope from poachers living on nearby Kome Island.[60] In the first three months of 1914, scientists G. D. Hale Carpenter and W. F. Fiske toured over 30 islands between Entebbe and Jinja.[61]

Sleeping sickness control actions created African-free natural environments. The depopulated islands became an important realm for colonial science and set an early precedent for the colonization of East Africa as environment. Africa without Africans was a place where colonialists forged identities as scientist-heroes as opposed to administrators. Theoretically, there were none of the distractions of inhabited areas—responding to Africans' needs and demands, or overtly creating and maintaining colonial relationships (except with the groups of accompanying African workers). Scientists could carry out pure research in these natural settings. This practice was an extension of the ideas of the colonial botanical garden and the game reserve, with colonial science adding the component of research.[62] The existence of these spaces, and scientists' research in them, articulated, justified, and reified the importance of science and ongoing scientific work.

For local Africans, the extent of scientific expeditions into infected areas brought the scientific rationale of depopulation into further question and further justified trespassing. The apparent exemption of white scientists and their African employees from sleeping sickness rules contradicted the rhetoric of strict environmental isolation. There was also a great deal of regular trespassing by local people. Since game flourished in what were now effectively game reserves, infected areas became increasingly valuable for fishing, hunting, and charcoal production as the absorption of displaced people put added pressure on resources in legal areas bordering closed lands. Local people emphasized the extent to which they regularly entered closed areas and remained healthy. Samuel Kinbya recounted that his father and uncles hunted in illegal areas where there had been little game before depopulation: "The times of going out hunting did not change. Before [depopulation] they left before dawn and returned after dark to look for animals in the early morning and evening. During the day they rested. After [depopulation] police were not out when it was dark. During the day they hid from the police. Most of them did not get the sickness."[63]

Inspection tours regularly found signs of trespassing. Sleeping sickness officers' inspection reports are rife with reports of illegal fishing camps, charcoal production sites, signs of hunting parties, and of canoes they discovered and destroyed. For fishers, the transportation and marketing of fresh fish was dangerous, so drying fish became the safest way to process catches. Fishers could leave hidden drying camps unattended for days while the fish dried. Once the fish were in legal area markets, it was difficult for the police to prove they were from Lake Victoria. Officials destroyed property but caught few transgressors.

The extent of colonial enforcement was extremely limited relative to the accessibility of the infected areas by land and water. The medical superintendent of the sleeping sickness camp at Busu in Busoga, J. M. Collyns, wrote in 1908 that "deserted lake side shambas are constantly visited by land and water. There is constant canoe traffic in all directions."[64] The winding shores and overgrown lands provided good hiding places. Mukeri Landing on Sigulu Island is an example of a landing established by fishers because of the sleeping sickness regulations. It cannot be seen from the open lake or the main island, and is only accessible by land by a small path through the swamp, and by water through a small opening in the papyrus. Asoman Wandoka, a former lake fisherman interviewed at Mukeri, recalled fishing in the 1920s:

We stayed in many new secret landings in the swamps, and moved only at night. These are still good places. We hid from the British doctors, then we hid from all the soldiers, now we hide from the revenue collectors. Whites patrolled with motorboats so it was dangerous to come. We would stay here for a few weeks, then take smoked fish back. When Sigulu was opened, I built a house here.

In response to questions about sleeping sickness, he said, "Some of us fell sick and died. But we fished. That is what we did. You belonged where you could earn a living at that time."[65] Colonial scientists saw infected areas as health risks for local people, as a means to environmental order, and as necessitating and creating spaces for research. For farmers and fishers, the value of these changing environments for food and material extraction outweighed legal and health risks, and the closed areas were considered products of the suspect motives and methods of colonial science.

SLEEPING SICKNESS CAMPS

Sleeping sickness controls also ordered the creation of medical camps for the segregation and treatment of people infected with trypanosomes. Africans' reactions to sleeping sickness controls were related, as well, to the reputation of these spaces the British created for the sick. Coinciding with the beginning of removals in late 1906, sleeping sickness authorities constructed four sleeping sickness camps alternately referred to by colonial officials as segregation and concentration camps. The Sleeping Sickness Commission established camps at Buwanuka in Busiro in November 1906, at Bussu in Busoga in July 1907, then later that year at Kyetume in Chagwe and on Bugala Island in the Sesses. Missionaries and colonial officials reported that local people had their own strategies of segregating sleeping sickness victims—abandoning them in the bush to die of disease, starvation, or be killed by animals.[66] Colonial camps, in contrast, would more humanely serve the needs of both ordered society and science. They were to provide semiquarantined care for the ill, administer experimental drug cures, and investigate the disease through patient observation and testing. Bsweri Kaboli and Nambula Bigogo, who both grew up near the Bussu camp in Busoga, recalled that families did not abandon the sick in the forest to die alone, but sometimes hid the sick outside homesteads to protect them from being found by colonial officials and sent to sleeping sickness camps.[67]

Sleeping sickness scientists chose campsites outside of declared infected areas, but near enough for patient access, and removed from colonial and African centers. Forced, local labor and patients constructed the camps. The original idea was that patients would be accompanied by "healthy relations who would, by their labours, provide food and necessaries for the sufferer."[68] But relatives often brought only the most severe and advanced cases to camp and then abandoned them there. Families and friends considered the camps a last resort when home care had failed and a final destination for the sick.[69] A story from near the Bussu camp location was that patients were often too sick to walk, so people would carry them by litter and leave them at the camp entrance. The sick often died waiting in line to be processed and admitted. Camp workers then buried bodies in a large trench grave dug just outside the camp.[70]

The reputation of camp conditions and patient treatment there led people to avoid medical examinations, the sick to resist internment, and people to abandon the sick in camps. Official death counts in the camps averaged 25 percent annually, with 800 of 6,600 admitted patients still alive by 1910.[71] A popular sense of the camps was that "everyone died there."[72] A colonial report on the Bussu camp noted, "The unsophisticated natives associate the place mainly with the idea of death and shun it accordingly."[73] In 1920 people passing through Entebbe on their way back to the Lake Victoria islands refused to be given gland exams. They knew that exams might lead to the end of their repatriation and to internment in sleeping sickness camps.[74]

This reputation, along with famine in 1908, made it difficult for the camps to carry out original plans of purchasing local food supplies and relying on family members for patient care.[75] In response to this problem, camp officials planted sweet potatoes and bananas, as camp administrations maneuvered to maintain sufficient material support for patients and not become increasingly dependent on the colonial budget. But patients resisted farming at the camps: "They say they are going to die, so why grow food for others."[76] To attract patients and promote patient cooperation, camp administrators issued them mattresses, bark-cloth, cooking pots, and sometimes blankets. Practical revisions of camp administration in the case of camp farms and material supplies isolated the camps from local people and from the interference of other colonial interest groups.

Camp isolation and self-sufficiency allowed scientific authorities to apply medical strategies relatively independent from patients' families and communities. Colonial concerns about humane treatment were balanced against scientific necessity—always with the ultimate good of the native as justifying anchor. Disease treatment, though not conditions, was similar to that in hospitals in Europe. Doctors gave patients daily examinations, regular cerebrospinal fluid taps (lumbar punctures), and lymphatic gland punctures to test for trypanosome concentrations.[77] Aides administered experimental regimes of drug injections between the shoulder blades. These included Atoxyl (an arsenic-based drug) combined with strychnine or mercury, Atoxyl alone, and mercury alone. The camps communicated on the types, amounts, and frequency of drug injections each was trying: four-tenths of a gram every 20th and 21st day, or every 10th and 11th day, or gradual dose increases on these days to seven-tenths of a gram, or the German commission's recommendation of one gram repeated every 15th and 16th day.[78] The scientists noted possible side effects of toxicity such as convulsions, blindness, and death but considered them necessary risks in the face of certain death. Sleeping sickness doctors performed immediate postmortems on the dead and recorded their findings to complete comprehensive case studies for Royal Society reports.

Treatment was combined with enthusiastic publication of papers and ac-cumulation of records that established the camp scientists on the frontiers of knowledge and the subjugation of tropical disease. Scientists recorded detailed case studies documenting various drug-use schemes on humans, for example, followed by reports of the same drug experiments being carried out simul-taneously on monkeys, rats, and dogs.[79] By 1910 the Sleeping Sickness Com-mission of the Royal Society in London had published 10 report compilations from Uganda.

Camp officials negotiated the issue of force in their favor as well. The sleeping sickness commissioner initially advocated forced detention for all Africans suspected of infection, but he was convinced (by a field scientist) that the camps would be more popular if people were allowed to come of their own accord.[80] Self-admittance left the issue of force up to local chiefs who were directed to "advise" infected people to report to sleeping sickness camps. In a political climate where chiefs gained favor from the colonial state through a reputation as being cooperative, this policy informally condoned force. Chief Skeibob, whose lands bordered Kyetume camp, reported that although he had been directed not to use force, deserters were difficult to return. In particular, "Buvuma people in Kyetume camp are stubborn and go back [to Buvuma] on their own accord. But now as his Excellency has ordered us to return them we will persuade them to return by their own wish. We will tell them that even if they are better they have still got the disease and we will tell them to return to be cured."[81] By 1909 a Dangerous Disease Ordinance from the governor resolved this ambiguity, making it illegal for those directed to camps by a medical officer not to go or for patients to leave without authorization.[82]

There was the further complication of how resistance was perceived in such scientific environments. Camp definitions of patient needs reinforced the needs of research experimentation. For patients, internment meant they were left for dead by their communities, legally imprisoned for being ill, and reg-ularly tested and injected by white doctors. Then camp rules segregated the sick by sex and had them forcibly bathed and deloused. Patients had a range of responses to such treatment from riot to desertion to despair.[83] There were also patient suicides and "lunatic" vandalism:

The average advanced case is a harmless imbecile, but violent mania is sometimes seen. Sixty-one patients in all have had to be isolated and restrained in our various camps. Each of our camps is now provided with a special lunatic annex to which violent cases can be sent. Our camp buildings are, of course, only roofed with dried grass; on two occasions lunatics have succeeded in setting fire to the camps, and have done a great deal of damage. Native warders are in charge of them both day and night. Violent patients are handcuffed, but there is always the danger that some patient may become suddenly maniacal, and burn down the whole camp.[84]

Mania is a symptom of late-stage trypanosome infection. But in Uganda in the early twentieth century, the distinctions within colonial science between African responses to science and African symptoms of sleeping sickness were vague. As late as 1956 a colonial report on sleeping sickness argued that mania might be part of a primitive psychological response to the disease, as opposed to a universal symptom: "Mania may occasionally occur because the African in the bush, with his background of witchcraft, will react to any illness quite differently from the European."[85] For camp authorities, as well as scientific interests in Uganda, mania was a tidy analysis of all patient violence and a justification for coercion as medically necessary.

CONCLUSION

Sleeping sickness control policies in colonial Uganda in the early twentieth century meant distinctly different things to Ganda elites, Ganda peasants, Soga and Buvuma farmers and fishers, and to British colonialists. Each group coordinated, as much as it could, colonial disease control to accord with its own political and economic interests. For British colonial administrators, the sleeping sickness control plan fit with the policy of informal control, protected a potentially valuable colonial labor force, and reflected colonial legitimacy as a morally necessary defense of human life against disease. For colonial scientists in particular, sleeping sickness control provided an important opportunity to assess certain scientific methods. Moreover a subtle, but inescapable, parallel was drawn between colonial designations of the most diseased places and colonial perceptions of the most politically resistant people. Colonial officers came to characterize the lake islands as difficult to order socially as well as environmentally. They identified islanders not only in view of their culture and economic activity but also merely by virtue of their location and their proximity to certain physical environments as diseased people.

For local Africans, there were both potential political and economic advantages and disadvantages in cooperating with the colonial state's policy of land alienation or population relocations. The meanings that elite and nonelite Africans assigned to the depopulation of lands depended on their status within the Buganda Kingdom and on their political identity as Ganda, Nyoro, Bavuma, Soga, or Sesse. In the minds of farmers and fishers, colonial policies could not alter their perception of disease and its relation to the environment. Colonial policies did transform some agricultural lands to forests, and farmers and fishers shifted their use of these lands accordingly. Local Africans considered the penalties of trespassing, along with the risks of sickness and other physical risks of working in forests or on water, when making decisions about their relationships to sleeping sickness control regulations.

NOTES

1. Bell, *Glimpses*, 164. At this date, only mainland depopulations had begun.

2. Interview with Samuel Kinbya, Luwanika, Busoga, December 30, 1993.

3. Five of six infected areas were reopened in 1924. In 1935, only the Kative infected area by Lake George and Lake Edward still existed. See Thomas and Scott, 342.

4. Letter from A. D. P. Hodges to District Commissioner Busoga, August, 1906, Secretariate Minute 874, Uganda National Archives (UNA), Entebbe.

5. Ibid.

6. Bell, *Glimpses*, 163–164.

7. Shula Marks and Neil Anderson, "Typhus and Social Control: South Africa: 1917–1950," and Rodney Sullivan, "Cholera and Colonialism in the Philippines, 1899–1903," in Macleod and Lewis. Also see David Arnold, "Smallpox and Colonial Medicine in Nineteenth Century India," I. J. Catanach, "Plague and the Tensions of Empire: India, 1896–1918," and Reynaldo C. Ileto, "Cholera and the Origins of the American Sanitary Order in the Philippines," in Arnold, *Imperial Medicine*.

8. Bell, *Glimpses*, 163.

9. Beck, *British Medical*, 43.

10. Letter from A. D. P. Hodges to District Commissioner Busoga, August, 1906, Secretariate Minute 874, UNA.

11. Ibid., 35; Bell, *Glimpses*, 163.

12. Entebbe Township Ordinance, 1906, Secretariat Minute 1099, UNA.

13. A. D. P. Hodges to District Commissioner Busoga, February 15, 1906, UNA; Soff, "A History of Sleeping Sickness," 94.

14. Chief Kweba and Chief Mbubi to the Governor, April, 1909, Secretariat Minute 396, UNA.

15. Letter from Kabaka Daudi Chwa to Corydon, April 8, 1921, UNA, quoted in Soff, "A History of Sleeping Sickness," 197.

16. Hesketh Bell, Introduction to A. C. H. Gray "Report on the Sleeping Sickness Camps, Uganda," 63.

17. Sleeping Sickness Report, December 1909, Secretariat Minute 584, UNA; David Bruce, "Sleeping Sickness in Uganda: Duration of the Infectivity of the Glossina palpalis after the Removal of the Lake Shore Population," *Reports of the Sleeping Sickness Commission of the Royal Society (RSSSCRS)*, X(1910), 56–57. A more recent scientific conclusion is that the disease-carrying ability does last the entirety of an infected tsetse fly's life and that the life span of the tsetse fly is 60 to 80 days. See Knight, 27.

18. Soff, "A History of Sleeping Sickness," 150.

19. Ibid., 196–198.

20. District Officer Tour Report, 1910, Secretariat Minute 1094, UNA.

21. Greig, 274; A. Hodges, "Report on Sleeping Sickness in Unyoro and Nile Valley," *RSSCRS*, VIII(1906), 86–99; A. G. Speke and E. B. Adams, 100–105.

22. Langlands, 18–32.

23. Interview with Bsweri Kaboli, Luwanika, Busoga, December 28, 1993; Soff, "A History of Sleeping Sickness," 119.

24. Interview with Samuel Kinbya, Wambeti, Busoga, December 30, 1993; Interview with Bsweri Kaboli, Luwanika, Bugosa, December 28, 1993; Interview with Jackson Bubolo, Bugoto, Iganga, November 11, 1993.

25. Medical Officer Report, 1908, Secretariat Minute 2015, UNA; Soff, "A History of Sleeping Sickness," 119.

26. Bell, Introduction to Gray, "Report on the Sleeping Sickness Camps, Uganda," 63.

27. Bell, *Glimpses*, 164. At this date, only mainland depopulations had begun.

28. Bell, Introduction to Gray, "Report on the Sleeping Sickness Camps, Uganda, December, 1906 to November, 1907," 63.

29. Sleeping Sickness Payment Report, 1908, Secretariat Minute 2015, UNA.

30. Ibid.

31. Hodges, *Explanatory Address*.

32. Interview with Jackson Bubolo, Bugoto, Iganda, November 11, 1993.

33. Hesketh Bell, "Report on the Measures Adopted for the Suppression of Sleeping Sickness in Uganda," Secretariat Minute 4990, 1909, UNA.

34. Interview with Bsweri Kaboli, Luwanika, Busoga, December 28, 1993. Numerous informants had personal memories of depopulations in 1941, and their discussions of the early century were history.

35. Sleeping Sickness Guard Report, 1911, Secretariat Minute 1094, UNA.

36. Ibid.

37. Medical Officer Report, 1908, Secretariat Minute 1614, UNA.

38. Soff, "A History of Sleeping Sickness," 152–155.

39. Chief Kweba and Chief Mbubi to the Governor, April, 1909, Secretariat Minute 396, UNA.

40. Resettlement Directive, 1911, Secretariat Minute 1814, UNA.

41. Interview with John Bubolo, Bugoto, Busoga, November 11, 1993.

42. Soff, "A History of Sleeping Sickness," 154.

43. Ibid., 158.

44. *Uganda Protectorate Medical and Sanitary Annual Report for 1913* (Entebbe, 1914), 23; *Uganda Protectorate Medical and Sanitary Annual Report for 1917* (Entebbe, 1918), 13.

45. "Uganda Fishing Ordinance of 1907," *Uganda Gazette*, 1907, and "Sleeping Sickness Rules Number 2, December, 1908," *Uganda Gazette*, 1908.

46. Soff, "A History of Sleeping Sickness," 151.

47. A. D. P. Hodges, *Sleeping Sickness Clearing Scheme* (Entebbe, 1911), 1.

48. Ibid., 4.

49. Soff, "A History of Sleeping Sickness," 21.

50. "Sleeping Sickness Rules (no. 2)," *Uganda Gazette*, 1909, UNA.

51. Sese Islands Tour Report, 1908, Secretariat Minute 1807, UNA.

52. *Uganda Protectorate Medical and Sanitary Report of 1938* (Entebbe, 1939), 39.

53. Sleeping Sickness Inspection Report, January 16, 1908, Secretariat Minute 72, UNA.

54. Sleeping Sickness Report, October 22, 1930, Busoga District Archives (BDA), Jinja.

55. Field Report, Assistant Sleeping Sickness Officier, Busoga, November 4, 1929, BDA.

56. *Uganda Gazette*, 1909, UNA. Landings with colonial spellings.

57. Interview with Samuel Kinbya, Wambeti, Busoga, December 30, 1993.

58. Inspection Report, Busoga, May, 1910, Secretariat Minute 1614, UNA.

59. Duke, 54–57; Carpenter, "Progress Report," 79–107.

60. Thomas and Scott, 399.

61. Carpenter, "Bionomics," 3–66.

62. Grove, *Green Imperialism*; Mackenzie, *Empire of Nature*.

63. Interview with Samuel Kinbya, Luwanika, Bosoga, December 30, 1993.

64. J. M. Collyns, Busu Sleeping Sickness Camp Report, October 24, 1908, Secretariat Minute 89, UNA.

65. Interview with Asoman Wandoka, Sigulu Island, Busoga, December 9, 1993.

66. Medical Officer's Report, 1909, Secretariat Minute 4990, UNA.

67. Interview with Bsweri Kaboli, Luwanika, Busoga, December 28, 1993; Interview with Nambula Bigogo, Bugoto, Busoga, November 11, 1993.

68. Gray, "Report on the Sleeping Sickness Camps, Uganda, and on the Medical Treatment of Sleeping Sickness Patients at the Segregation Camps, from December, 1906, to January, 1908," 70.

69. Interview with Samuel Kinbya, Luwanika, Busoga, December 30, 1993.

70. Group interview at trench grave site, Bussu, Busoga, November 29, 1993.

71. Gray, "Report on the Sleeping Sickness Camps, Uganda, December, 1906, to November, 1907," 71–78.

72. Interview with Samuel Kinbya, Wambeti, Busoga, December 30, 1993; Interview with Bsweri Kaboli, Luwanika, December 30, 1993.

73. Bell, Introduction to Gray, "Reports on the Sleeping Sickness Camps, Uganda," 66.

74. C. A. Wiggins, Principal Medical Officer, Uganda Department of Health and Sanitation, 1920, ZA, 64.

75. P. Nayenga, "Busoga in the era of Catastrophes 1898–1911," in B. A. Ogot, ed., *Ecology and History in East Africa* (Nairobi, 1979), 170–173.

76. Gray, "Report on the Sleeping Sickness Camps, Uganda, December, 1906, to November, 1907," 84.

77. Gray and Tulloch, 7–11.

78. Gray, "Report on the Sleeping Sickness Camps, Uganda," 90–91.

79. Gray and Tulloch.

80. Ibid., 66.

81. Chief Skeibob to Medical Officer, Kyetume Camp, 1907, Secretariat Minute 1627, UNA.

82. "Dangerous Disease Ordinance of April, 1909," *Uganda Gazette* (Entebbe, 1909).

83. For responses by Africans in sleeping sickness camps in the northern Belgian Congo see Lyons, 183–198.

84. Gray, 82–83.

85. *Sleeping Sickness, the Disease and Its Diagnosis* (Dar es Salaam, 1956), 4.

CHAPTER 4

The Shift to Tanganyika, 1920–1935

The territorial focus of British sleeping sickness control research and implementation shifted after World War I from Uganda to the new protectorate of Tanganyika. The British considered the epidemic crisis in Uganda ended by 1914, although controls and localized outbreaks continued there through the end of colonial rule. On the other hand, after World War I Tanganyika was a new protectorate in need of new mechanisms of colonial development and control for remote and impoverished populations. Beginning in the 1920s, tsetse control became an important part of British colonization in northwest Tanganyika in the areas that lay between Lake Victoria and Lake Tanganyika.

The British approach to sleeping sickness control in Tanganyika was different from control schemes in early colonial Uganda. A shift occurred away from focusing on disrupting the spread of the disease through emergency segregation to controlling the spread of tsetse. There was no major sleeping sickness epidemic in Tanganyika as there had been in Uganda, but colonial scientists reported massive and spreading fly infestations. In 1913 the German administration estimated that one-third of German East Africa was tsetse infested. In 1924 British scientists warned that tsetse were expanding rapidly into new areas and that three-quarters of the territory were threatened. British maps in 1937 showed tsetse occupying two-thirds of Tanganyika—nearly 200,000 square miles.[1] This was too much land for the administration to depopulate, as had been conceivable in Uganda. There was also no effective, centralized African state power to work through, as had been the case in Uganda. In further contrast to early visions of Uganda, the British saw northwest Tanganyika as environmentally desolate and politically disordered with little economic potential. They did not dream of robust and profitable peasant production, but of self-sufficient, stable, indirect rule and a steady flow of men to plantation wage employment.[2]

The British developed a three-part colonial strategy of tsetse control for the vastness and dispersed populations of northwest Tanganyika. Initially, they would block the spread of tsetse by resettling local people together in concentrated settlement areas. Control plans would concentrate African farmers and pastoralists with enough population density to create contiguous brush-free cultivation fronts without tsetse or the threat of tsetse infestation. Simultaneously, to defend the borders between tsetse and resettlement areas, sleeping sickness authorities planned to organize African male labor to clear brush into extensive networks of precise tsetse barriers completely free of human and tsetse trespass. Eventually, within stable, defensive sleeping sickness settlements, human populations would grow, and inhabitants would expand out to win land back from tsetse.[3]

Noticeably missing from this strategy was game destruction, a method of tsetse control that was proving successful in southern Africa and northern Uganda but was opposed by wildlife conservationists. The career and work of Charles Swynnerton, the first chief game warden in Tanganyika in 1919 and the first director of tsetse research in 1930, together with the history of the tsetse research station at Shinyanga, reflects the influence of conservationist ideology on British tsetse control.

Beginning in the 1920s, colonial experimentation and intervention in Tanganyika set standards for the rest of British colonial Africa. Scientists with experience in Tanganyika went on to direct tsetse-control programs in British West Africa, southern Africa, Kenya, and Uganda. Swynnerton's work reflects the transition from sleeping sickness control in Uganda at the turn of the century to tsetse control in Tanganyika in the 1920s and 1930s.

EUROPEAN IMAGES OF TANGANYIKA

> The flat central plains of Tanganyika with their endless covering of thorn bushes or slight trees might as well, so someone suggested, be written off altogether.
>
> M. MacMillan, 1952[4]

Nineteenth-century European reports of northwest Tanzanyika contrast greatly with reports of the fertility of Uganda, of the power of the Ganda state, and of Ugandans' intelligent and intensive use of their environments. European travelers and missionaries, many of the same that wrote about Uganda, emphasized instead vastness and desolation. After initial German colonial subjugation in the late nineteenth century, and then again after World War I, Europeans focused on the perceived emptiness of the landscape and poverty of its inhabitants. Colonialists employed these images to explain sleeping sickness and to justify sleeping sickness control depopulations, settlements, and forced labor for brush clearing.

Early colonial sources from the 1860s through the 1890s present an impression of environmental vastness to northwest Tanzanyika relative to human populations; they make connections between political decentralization, random settlement patterns, and mobility. Renowned nineteenth-century European explorers wrote of northwest Tanzanyika as vast, irregularly fertile, and randomly inhabited. Of his travels to the east of Lake Tanganyika in the 1870s, Joseph Thomson reported, "A more bleak and barren prospect as far as the eye could reach could hardly be conceived." He described lands to the southwest of Tabora as "poorly inhabited forest country" and the plateau of Ugogo east of Tabora as "burnt-up waterless deserts."[5] Richard Burton characterized his route west from the coast through "the tangled thickets of Ujiji" and the "barrens" of Usukuma.[6] According to Oscar Baumann, besides small villages near sources of water, "the rest of the land is thorny and open."[7] For Karl Weule, writing in 1909, central German East Africa "neither impresses us with the number and size of its trees, nor refreshes us with any shade whatever, nor presents the slightest variation in the eternal monotony that greets the traveler." He cautioned against Africa's reputation for natural exuberance: "See that the general public is more correctly informed as to the supposed fertility of Equatorial Africa, and so saved from forming extravagant notions of the brilliant future in store for our colonies."[8]

Colonial authors linked images of vast, open landscapes to the relationship Africans had with their lands. European visitors depicted Africans as mobile, often and easily changing locations. They mentioned abandoned villages and depopulated lands in Uzinza, Unyamwezi, and Uhehe caused by warfare and the slave trade.[9] Thomson wrote of the villages he visited, "There is probably not one now standing. Such is the evanescent nature of governments, people and villages in Africa."[10] These reports of settlement represented Africans both as having little control over and little investment in their environments. Franz Stuhlmann wrote that the Unyamwezi were unwise in their use of land and unskilled in their keeping of cattle. When they decided soil was exhausted, they simply moved to new land.[11]

European impressions of African transience were reinforced by descriptions of inconsequential architecture. Baumann observed, "Often the huts are so light, that a person without difficulty can carry it from one place to another."[12] European travelers in the nineteenth century tended to perceive Africans as moving through landscapes but not affecting nature in a long-term way. In the 1880s Edward Hore described Unyamwezi in his diary: "Alternate forest and open glades with scattered bushes—almost level—but rough ground over hard baked mud; footprints of man and game."[13] Like wildlife, Africans left only passing traces on the environment.

European observers connected the aesthetic deficiencies of these landscapes to the cultural and political deficiencies of local residents. Europeans reported a region of interminable small squabbles, theft, and petty local responses to new people and ideas.[14] In marked contrast to descriptions of Uganda, European missionaries, naturalists, and officials described Sukuma and Zinza dwellings as dirty and inconsequential. While Paul Kollman described Uganda as "peopled by a race which is entitled to our special attention, in consequence of its high degree of civilization," he reported that the people to the east of Lake Victoria were warlike and lived in small, dirty huts in autonomous villages without chiefs.[15] Colonial officers complained of the total lack of political authority. Reports from 1924 called Zinza rulers "utterly untrustworthy and useless" and the Zinza people "unsettled tribal communities."[16] As late as 1960 anthropologist Audrey Richards wrote of the Zinza, "The whole area is poor and 'backward' and the lack of assimilated European values is very marked."[17]

The British assumed control of German East Africa beginning in 1917, inheriting, as well, images of impoverishment and desolation. Donald Cameron, the British colonial governor of Tanganyika from 1925 to 1931, emphasized that Tanganyika was "with a somewhat cruel climate for the agriculturalist" and not suitable for white settlement: "I saw six harvests in the Territory, and one only of those was fairly good. [I]n some localities the people had gone into the woods as a matter of course to dig up roots and endeavor to find other precarious means of keeping themselves from starvation."[18] He mentions the "miserable condition" of Biharamulo.[19] While traveling outside Musoma, Cameron saw "wretched people" so desperate they tried to steal an antelope from a lion to feed themselves.[20]

Such images informed and reinforced the initial post–World War I position of Tanganyika in the broader British colonial agenda. Even before World War I, the British were incapable of developing all their possessions.[21] Colonies other than Tanganyika presented much more potentially profitable possibilities. The colonial office sought to establish indirect rule in Tanganyika and to minimize colonial investments in the colony. The perceived poverty and desolation of Tanganyika provided the British with both an excuse and an incentive to marginalize it within the colonial empire.

European observers' agendas also preselected environmental impressions. Many of the popular European books about Tanganyika from the early twentieth century were hunting and farming stories. Texts such as L. Von Brandis's *German Hunt on the Victoria Nyanza*, Hans Behrends's *Plains Wanderer: From my Farming and Hunting Life in East Africa*, and Joyce Boyd's *My Farm in Lion Country*, depicted African environments and people in terms of the particular interests of the colonial authors.[22] Most German and British colonial officials hunted, and hunting stories were popular in Europe. Tales of hunting focused on wildlife environments distant from human settlement. And white farms also were often geographically separated from African cultivation areas. Joyce Boyd wrote of the view from her farm near Arusha in the 1920s: "In every direction, for miles, the forest densely stretched, with beyond the open country rolling desolately away to the sapphire hills in the far distance. No sign of human habitation of civilization could be seen."[23] The occupations of colonial observers affected how they perceived lands and local people.

Europeans' environmental observations about Tanzanyika illustrate Mary Louise Pratt's discussion of the "monarch-of-all-I-survey scene" as a mechanism of European colonial representation. According to Pratt, the esthetic deficiencies of African landscapes "suggest a need for social and material intervention by the home culture."[24] Europeans emphasized Africans' transience in the apparently uninhabited vastness of the territory. In the emerging colonial logic of environmental imperialism, if Africans had few permanent connections to the land, they also had few claims to it. By failing to recognize local African strategies to control nature, Europeans could figuratively, and sometimes literally, write Africans out of African environments.

ENVIRONMENT AND HISTORY IN NORTH-CENTRAL TANZANYIKA

European depictions of African transience, bare-subsistence production systems, poverty, and lack of political order were important bases for British tsetse-control policies in Tanganyika. The period from 1870 to 1920 was one of severe socioeconomic and environmental disruption. As in Uganda, African actions affected European perceptions of environment and disease. Nineteenth- and early-twentieth-century African and colonial histories informed where tsetse were and the context of colonial sleeping sickness control. The economic and political changes in the nineteenth century included extensive slave raiding, Ngoni invasions from the south, and Nyamwezi empire building along major caravan routes to the Indian Ocean coast. Rinderpest, German colonialization, and World War I brought further environmental and economic destabilization.

Colonial texts from the late nineteenth century provide some evidence about the political and socioeconomic organization of people living between Lake Victoria and Lake Tanganyika. However, it is difficult to know how much Africans' responses to political change and ecological collapse during this time transformed local people's relationships with their environments, and how much continuity existed from earlier conditions.[25] The large number of separate language groups involved also makes any generalizations problematic. At the turn of the twentieth century, northwest Tanzanyika was composed of fragmented, small political units with no centralized political organization.[26] The Sukuma, the largest and most centralized group in the area, were approximately 40 multichiefdom states.[27] There is evidence of nineteenth-century intercommunity and interchiefdom conflict resulting in early European reports of abandoned, destroyed villages and depopulated areas.[28]

The Sukuma were agropastoralists. Cattle played an important economic role for them, and parts of the area were heavily stocked. But the Sukuma did not closely integrate cattle and farming and could adjust to the loss of stock without major cultural disruptions.[29] The Zinza, Ha, and most other groups in northwest Tanzania, in contrast, kept few livestock. They practiced extensive agriculture with no systematic crop rotation or fallow. When soil was exhausted, farmers switched to other plots.[30] Banana plantations were uncommon, and primarily maize, cassava, and millet composed people's diets. People near bodies of water consumed fish as an important protein source. There were few strong institutions of land ownership or farmer clientage but rather conditional occupations according to land use. Landholders inherited holdings but did not subdivide them. Elites were the symbolic custodians of land and they made tribute demands for labor and goods.[31]

Families and individuals moved between villages and chiefdoms for better land or to avoid conflicts with neighbors, elites, slave raiders, and African and European invaders. The structure of Sukuma communities easily integrated strangers. Village leaders would assign new settlers vacant land upon their arrival.[32] Local people had open access to noncultivated land for grazing, hunting, and honey and firewood collection.[33] The Sukuma did not specifically define boundaries between villages, chiefdoms, and homesteads, and occupied areas were separated by tracts of unsettled land.[34] John Ford emphasizes the importance of these wilderness borders (*Grenzwildnes*) in his analysis of African relationships to endemic sleeping sickness.[35]

Along with histories of mobility and limited productivity in this area, there is evidence of shifting frontiers. People claimed farms in unpopulated areas outside established political authority by virtue of clearing the land, and groups expanded and contracted territorially over time.[36] Beginning in the 1930s, Sukuma migrated in large numbers west across Lake Victoria's Smith Sound into Zinza areas of Geita District. In 1950, four of seven chiefdoms in Geita were Sukuma dominated.[37] The British made the eastern Zinza kingdoms part of the Sukuma Federation in 1950.[38]

Zinza living just south of Lake Victoria and west of the Sukuma have a nineteenth-century history of migrations from the south and west generating cultural mixing and conflict. There was raiding by Ngoni and Nyamwezi in the area beginning in the mid-nineteenth century, and dynastic wars. In the colonial period, Zinza in Geita and Biharamulo lived together with Ha, Nyabo, and Rinda populations. More centralized Zinza kingdoms existed further west in Biharamulo as a southern extension of the interlacustrine state systems of central Africa. But soil and rainfall south of the lake did not support permanent settlement around banana plantations, and the area remained a political and environmental frontier for the Zinza and Sukuma.[39]

Germany claimed the colony of German East Africa in 1885. German intervention was most pervasive toward the Indian Ocean coast. Emin Pasha, working for the German colonial administration after leaving Equatoria, led a German military force through Unyamwezi and Usukuma to Lake Victoria in 1890. He founded military stations at Mwanza and Bukoba. German forces based at these stations intervened in local politics and fought in numerous minor military engagements through World War I.[40] Although the German colonial state consolidated power more effectively beginning in 1900 in some eastern, northeastern, and central parts of the colony and in the area around Bukoba, there was little German government to the south and east of Lake Victoria through 1918.[41] Germans attempted some inland plantation production of coffee, cotton, rubber, and sisal. Local people resisted colonial taxation and the mandatory growing of cash crops. The Maji Maji Rebellion from 1905 to 1907 began as resistance to mandatory cotton growing. The rebellion focused in the Songea District to the northeast of Lake Nyasa and resulted in the massive loss of African lives and environmental devastation due to the German military's scorched-earth policy. Socioeconomic devastation and loss of life in the colony continued through various campaigns of World War I fought between German and Allied armies. This 60-year history of conflict and dislocation probably promoted the spread of tsetse and endemic sleeping sickness.

The British-occupied German East Africa beginning in 1917 and annexed the colony in 1922 as a mandate from the League of Nations, renaming it *Tanganyika*. The British government was interested in the protectorate primarily as a political investment in regional security to avoid possible future threats to Indian Ocean commerce and communications and as part of the "Cape to Cairo" vision, and not as a potentially valuable economic possession.[42] The British considered Tanganyika as an impoverished part of the British colonial sphere. Private investment was minimal when the state auctioned off German sisal estates.[43] The protectorate was subordinate in the 1920s to Kenya through customs arrangements and through the political and economic centers of Nairobi and Mombasa.[44] There was both a lack of white interest in settlement and an official interest in discouraging settlers in order to avoid having to develop the infrastructures and making the investments necessary to promote and support a settler economy. The overt agenda of the British colonial office and the Tanganyikan colonial state was to establish colonial rule through existing African political systems and to promote African self-sufficient economic development. The colonial office appointed Donald Cameron as governor in part because of his 17 years of administrative experience with indirect rule in Nigeria.[45]

As with German rule, the British colonization of the area between Lake Victoria and Lake Tanganyika was minimal relative to other parts of the colony. Europeans had little interest in settlement or plantation production here. The Sukuma were an important source of labor for plantations in north and central Tanganyika.[46] Beginning in the 1930s, some small-scale gold mining developed in Geita and Mwanza, and the Sukuma development scheme promoted peasant cotton production. But even after the Colonial Welfare and

Development Act of 1940 began financing long-term colonial development plans, colonial economic development and presence in the area was minimal.

Tsetse were endemic in northwest Tanganyika, and the location of tsetse reflected and affected settlement patterns, pastoralism, and mobility. Local people either avoided or maintained low-level contact with tsetse. Controlled exposure to trypanosomes might have developed resistance in human and cattle populations although scientists continue to dispute this possibility. But local people and cattle in Tanganyika did coexist with tsetse. Tsetse and trypanosomiasis kept cattle populations low and localized but did not prevent cattle keeping.[47] Whether controlling trypanosomiasis through avoidance or through limited exposure, local people understood the relationship between contact with tsetse and sickness in cattle and they modified their environments and their relationship to their environments in response to tsetse and trypanosomiasis. These systems of trypanosomiasis control often broke down during the violence and disruptions of the nineteenth and early twentieth centuries.[48]

African responses to colonization and ecological crises at the turn of the century influenced European perceptions of environment and African relationships to the land and tsetse. Certainly Sukuma and Zinza resisted colonization with increased mobility, moving away from colonial building projects and administrative centers. German cash-crop plantations, forced-labor demands, and an emerging colonial economy created new patterns of labor migration.[49] Although the Lake Victoria basin was marginal to the German plantation system, the Sukuma were an important source of migrant labor, in part because of their long-standing involvement in the long-distance caravan trade. Much of the early German colonial labor force was former caravan trade carriers transformed into migrant plantation labor.[50] The absence of Sukuma men from Sukuma villages promoted agricultural and pastoral decline leading to the expansion of tsetse brush. A missionary observed in 1912, "Abandoned or half-empty and decaying villages can be met everywhere; everywhere are the signs of old cultivation."[51]

Zinza mobility was promoted by the German construction of the central railroad between Dar es Salaam and Kigoma completed in 1914. European-manufactured iron hoes flooded the market and undermined Zinza iron smelting.[52] During World War I, the Germans drafted both Sukuma and Zinza men as porters and soldiers.[53] Colonial reports linked labor migration to immiserisation and depopulation. The impoverishment of the areas promoted further male out-migration. Sukuma fled German labor demands to build the Tabora-Mwanza Road in 1903, and the Germans reported the area as wilderness.[54] According to European authors, conflict in the mid-nineteenth century promoted settlement on high ground near Lake Victoria in fortified villages.[55] Colonial texts argue people reassumed authentic settlement patterns with the coming of colonial peace—they dispersed out of defensive villages into isolated homesteads (supposedly becoming more vulnerable to sleeping sickness in the process). Alfred Ishaka contradicts this argument: "People might move away from the village if there were difficulties with neighbors, or if they felt chiefs were not treating them fairly. Then they moved away because in the villages whites demanded taxes and took people away to work."[56] Sukuma and Zinza also responded to German military pacification beginning in the early 1890s through the Maji Maji Rebellion, and the grain, meat, and labor requisitions of World War I with out-migration. African mobility away from colonial outposts and work sites left Europeans with visions of uninhabited environmental desolation.

Early colonial violence and ecological collapse were interlinked tragedies in German East Africa.[57] Disease and famine made up components of the cycle. Animals carrying rinderpest entered in 1891, destroying livestock and game. Smallpox, sand fleas, and locust devastated large parts of the area throughout the decade. German colonial officials described deserted villages and empty lands. Baumann wrote of sand fleas, "Whole villages had died out on account of this vexation."[58] On the effects of the rinderpest on the Masai east of Lake Victoria, he wrote, "No human being could now be seen."[59] Baumann predicted demographic collapse: "The population of Unyamwezi has declined enormously and will soon disappear completely."[60] Germans wrote of depopulations and population dispersions into the bush. Von Lettow-Vorbeck observed of Singida District in 1914, "We passed through fertile districts which were completely forsaken by the inhabitants, but which were known to have been occupied even in the previous year. They had simply moved away, had settled somewhere else."[61] The German colonial newspaper, *Kolonialblatt*, stated simply, "The local people have left their villages and moved into the bush."[62] The loss of crops, animals, and labor weakened people's abilities to fend off famine and resist disease thus resulting in further losses.

World War I exacerbated the ecological crisis with massive grain, meat, and labor requisitions by both the Germans and Allies through 1918. In the central regions of Dodoma, Kondoa, and Singida, war combined with failed November rains to bring on three years of severe famine. In Ugogo, Greg Maddox estimates 30,000 of the total population of 150,000 died during this famine.[63] Smallpox again became widespread, and the Spanish influenza pandemic struck in 1918. As Africans moved away from European power and from European-fostered disease and environmental disruption, Europeans naturalized depopulated areas as wilderness and colonized the land now without people.

AFRICAN KNOWLEDGE AND THE POLITICS OF CONSERVATION

The conservationist-based approaches to tsetse control pursued by Charles Swynnerton were the result of a European understanding of Tanganyika as wilderness neglected by Tanganyikans. At the beginning of his career in Tanganyika, Swynnerton wrote, "There is no local demand for liberation from tsetse. The native has grown up with the situation. Owing to the fact just stated and the size and variety of the problem, this territory is ideal for that unhurried, scientific and thorough experimentation which will give us the real solution of the tsetse problem."[64] The scale and structure of research at Shinyanga reflected British images of Tanganyikan landscapes and Africans' place in these landscapes. Because the British considered so much of Tanganyika overrun by tsetse, or in threat of being overrun, tsetse control was an important component to the British colonial occupation of this part of the territory.

Swynnerton was not formally trained as a scientist. He was the son of a colonial chaplain in India and had studied natural history in England. In 1897 at the age of 19, he went to Natal for work. Swynnerton managed a farm until 1918 in Southern Rhodesia with Guy Marshall. Marshall later became head of the Imperial Bureau of Entomology and, along with Swynnerton, a member of the 1927 Tsetse Fly Committee.[65] Swynnerton's primary interests during this time were in hunting and natural science. In 1918 the Mozambique Company offered Swynnerton a three-month contract to survey tsetse fly behavior and habitat in the North Mossurise territory of Portuguese East Africa, not far from his farm in Southern Rhodesia. The company was suffering heavy cattle losses to nagana and hoped Swynnerton's research would help them develop ways to protect their profits. He published his North Mossurise tsetse research in 1921 in the *Bulletin of Entomological Research*. The long article, 80 pages with photographs and maps, brought together zoological, geological, climatic, and botanical observations and African oral evidence.[66]

Swynnerton became the first chief game warden of Tanganyika in 1919, and this appointment put him in a powerful position to influence tsetse-control policy. His experience and interests influenced the administration to make tsetse fly research and tsetse-infested land reclamation the responsibility of the tsetse division of the Game Department.[67] In 1921 the colonial office placed him in charge of tsetse research in the protectorate, and in 1922, in response to the Maswa sleeping sickness outbreak, the colonial office accepted Swynnerton's plans for tsetse control combining depopulations of tsetse-infested areas with creating barriers to the spread of tsetse through brush clearing.

The major debate at this time about tsetse control was over game destruction, and Swynnerton situated himself in this controversy on the side of conservation. White-settler game destruction was a nineteenth-century method for opening up pastures that some Europeans also believed controlled the spread of tsetse. The theory of game destruction was that game were either a reservoir for trypanosomes or carried tsetse flies, or both. The eradication of game meant cattle could safely move into an area and would then quickly graze and trample down tsetse bush to drive out any remaining tsetse. Colonial administrations, beginning in 1901 in the Natal and Southern Rhodesia, responded to white-settler demands for land with policies of unrestricted game shooting as nagana control. Through the 1960s in parts of Zimbabwe, Zambia, South Africa, and Malawi, settlers and game department hunters destroyed huge populations of game, making some species rare.[68]

Western conservation as a political force grew as a reaction to game destruction. John Mackenzie has traced the conflict between elite hunting interests and some colonial scientists and missionaries over this issue. Elite British hunting interests in Africa founded a preservationist lobby group, the Society for the Preservation of the Fauna of the Empire (SPFE) in 1903. This group quickly became a powerful political-pressure group and included high-ranking colonial officials and members of the colonial office and colonial scientific societies. It actively opposed game destruction as tsetse control. When the Interdepartmental Committee on Sleeping Sickness met for the first time in 1914, 6 of its 16 members were active conservationists.[69] This committee established the direction of sleeping sickness control in British East Africa in favor of the conservationists for the next 30 years.

In Uganda and Malawi, missionaries and the colonial state were interested in promoting African production and criticized game conservation as resulting in the destruction of villages and crops. Beginning in 1905 colonial administrators in Uganda argued, in particular, that buffalo, hippos, and elephants invaded fields, killed numerous local farmers, and that hunting regulations, therefore, should not protect these species.[70] In Tanganyika ideas for game preservation overlapped with images of the protectorate as containing abundant game in vast depopulated areas. Conservationists argued that game protection would not be socioeconomically disruptive for Africans. Missionary advocates of game destruction in Tanganyika, in contrast, argued that game protection would further impoverish Africans.[71]

The debate about game destruction was a contentious and much-discussed topic in southern Africa in Swynnerton and Marshall's circle of white hunters and settlers, and game destruction was important to Swynnerton's research in North Mossurise. In his 1921 article, Swynnerton praised Ngoni practices of bush clearing through burning and controlled settlement as effective tsetse controls. He argued, however, that Ngoni game destruction did not affect the spread of tsetse. According to Swynnerton, game was important only in the transportation of flies. Game destruction did not eliminate tsetse, but concentrated fly populations in specific areas. His position was that tsetse-control policies needed to separate people and livestock from wildlife by controlling human and game movements. At the Imperial Entomological conferences in 1925 and 1930, and until his death in Tanganyika in 1938, Swynnerton argued that the wholesale destruction of game needed to limit tsetse fly expansion was impractical and that experimentation with a combination of other kinds of environmental control would produce more effective results.

A basis of paternalist colonial interventions, such as disease control, in Africa was colonialists' belief that they understood African actions, African environments, and African problems better than Africans did. They maintained this position by prioritizing scientific method above African practice. The language, logic, organization, methods, and values of colonial sleeping sickness control were all informed by the overarching authority of science. As scientific practice, colonial sleeping sickness control was, by definition, superior to African control and better served Africans whether they recognized it or not. It was important to the ideology of colonial legitimacy that Africans did not accumulate empirical evidence or act scientifically, no matter the results.

In early colonial texts there was an acknowledgment and admiration of African knowledge and ideas about fly control.[72] Livingston discussed how he relied on African knowledge about tsetse areas to keep his cattle and oxen alive. He told of African game destruction and cattle fumigation as African methods of tsetse control.[73] In 1902 Franz Stuhlmann argued the important connection between local knowledge of tsetse areas and the economic viability of the colony.[74] European observers mentioned human excrement, lion fat, and herbal smears as other African methods of tsetse control.[75] In 1908 the German Bishop Spreiter wrote from German East Africa, "The Wachenzi often know more about these things than we highly educated Europeans."[76] Charles Swynnerton based his ideas about clearing and depopulation in part on his understanding of Ngoni practices in North Mossurise.

Swynnerton acknowledged the potential effectiveness of some African tsetse-control practices, but argued they were not rationally carried out. Ngoni resettlement was brutal and nonparticipatory, and random and uncontrolled African brush-burning was potentially counterproductive. Within a modernist discourse, scientific methods were superior to African methods because scientists proved the effects of controls in controlled research and through scientific observation, explained them in scientific language, and controlled them with a rational and geometrical plan. Although African understandings of environment and African actions might seem like good disease control, there was no evidence that they were scientifically derived. In colonialist discussions, unscientific African judgements and actions necessitated sleeping sickness control in the first place, and all African opposition to control policies was unscientific and illegitimate.

EARLY COLONIAL CONTROLS

Charles Swynnerton began resettlement and clearing experiments in the Maswa area near the Simiyu River in Shinyanga District in 1922. There was evidence of a sharp increase in the number of sleeping sickness victims in the area. With initial fly surveys in 1923 to 1925, Swynnerton showed the extent and speed of tsetse spread and human depopulation in the area, of epidemic rates of infection, and the need for drastic intervention. He was also attracted to the Shinyanga area because it was infested with four species of tsetse: *G. palpalis*, *G. morsitans*, *G. pallipides*, and *G. swynnertoni*. H. Stiebel, the district commissioner of the Lake Province, also lobbied Swynnerton to begin his work in Shinyanga to promote Sukuma political unity. Stiebel believed resettling parts of Shinyanga that Africans had depopulated because of tsetse would promote Sukuma unity under the chief of Shinyanga.[77] In contrast to the scale of the Uganda epidemic, during the Maswa epidemic from 1922 to 1938, medical officers identified a total of 564 sleeping sickness cases, peaking in 1925 with 108 cases.[78]

Under Swynnerton's direction in 1922, colonial officers ordered 5,000 people to evacuate to the periphery of the epidemic area. From 1926 through 1928, officers organized communal brush clearing to create further tsetse-free areas for settlement.[79] Moving people to the borders of a defined tsetse area created congestion on the margins and tensions with people already living in these areas.

Colonial officials in Biharamulo, Uha, Geita, and Kahama Districts, farther to the southwest of Lake Victoria, faced the problem of complete tsetse infestation. It was impossible to pull people back from fly areas because tsetse were everywhere. District officials tried to resettle and contain people in specific, brush-cleared locations, islands of settlement surrounded by supposedly depopulated fly areas. Resettlement became a massive undertaking in these districts in the late 1920s, with 60 settlements in place by 1934, and tens of thousands of men clearing brush. According to Kjekshus and based on census figures, colonial officials resettled 43 percent of the total population of Kahama District and 41 percent of Biharamulo.[80]

Colonial officials did not directly manage depopulation or resettlement, but issued directives to local elite to pull their people back behind a certain road or to one side of a geographic landmark. In the 1920s there were no official guidelines for the implementation of depopulation or for the form of resettlement, and control policies were haphazard depending on local conditions, colonial personnel, African elite, and local residents. In 1930 sleeping sickness surveyors found infected people in Geita, and from 1934 to 1936, resettled 5,400 people into six geographically defined sleeping sickness settlements.[81] In the late 1920s local officials organized communal male labor to sheer clear five 6-square-mile blocks 70 miles south of Tabora. They ordered local people into these blocks late in the dry season, where new residents first built new homes, then planted new fields. When planting was complete, officials allowed them to transport grain reserves from their former homesteads to the new villages. Medical officers gave residents routine exams to monitor for sleeping sickness infections.[82]

TSETSE RESEARCH AT SHINYANGA

Models for resettlement and brush clearing emanated primarily from the staff working at the Department of Tsetse Research headquarters and research station at Shinyanga. In 1930 Swynnerton resigned from the Game Department to form a new department, establishing its headquarters in a German fort at Old Shinyanga. In addition to being well-infested, Shinyanga was a relatively remote site with no competing colonial development interests such as mining or plantations. This isolation meant Swynnerton could operate independently. It was also near Maswa, so he could continue with his research and control work there. The department headquarters was well situated to pursue its mission of reclaiming fly-infested lands for productive use. Visitors' views of depopulated bush surrounding the station reinforced their impressions of how necessary and important the station's work was.

The direction, methods, and scope of research reflected the understandings colonial officials in Tanganyika had of African environments and of Africans' places in those environments. Swynnerton had environmental control over the entire Shinyanga District, as well as over parts of Kahama District to the west—totaling over 4,000 square miles. British assumptions were that the extent of tsetse infestation in Tanganyika justified research on this scale. Also, because the problem of tsetse in Tanganyika extended over such vast and supposedly desolate areas, with wandering game populations and people, colonial scientists justified large-scale experiments as necessary to achieve results applicable to large infested areas.

The history of research at Shinyanga also shows the importance of colonial science in legitimizing colonial policy. Colonial scientists in the Tsetse Research Department had extensive powers and freedoms to conduct wide-ranging projects. In 1929 the department had 14 European staff, and by 1939, it had 26.[83] Shinyanga became a world-renowned center of tsetse research. Scientists from the Tanganyikan Department of Tsetse Research, including entomologists, botanists, and zoologists who worked for Swynnerton, went on to direct tsetse-control schemes in Kenya, Uganda, Northern Rhodesia, and Nigeria.[84] Experiments at Shinyanga were the models for environmental intervention to control tsetse fly and sleeping sickness throughout British Africa after 1930 and, on the most massive scale, in Tanganyika.

By 1933 the Tsetse Research Department headquarters and research station at Shinyanga consisted of 13 irregularly shaped blocks encompassing 800 square miles of African-free nature. After 1945 the department created 4 new blocks adding over 600 more square miles of alienated land for research. Block sizes ranged from 4 to 100 square miles (see figure 4.1).[85] Tsetse officials tried to strictly control fly, animal, and human access in and out of the blocks. They considered the blocks to represent on a small, experimental scale what might be done to huge regions of Tanganyika. Researchers used the blocks as control areas and for experiments in clearing, game-fly relations, tsetse behavior, and habitat observation and, after World War II, for experiments in insecticide use, game destruction, and crossbreeding sterile tsetse. Tanganyikan workers counted animal and fly populations and charted movements. Researchers tried to separate animal species and drive certain species in and out of tsetse areas to observe the effects of contact and separation.[86]

Figure 4.1
Map of Shinyanga Research Station, Tanganyika, 1951

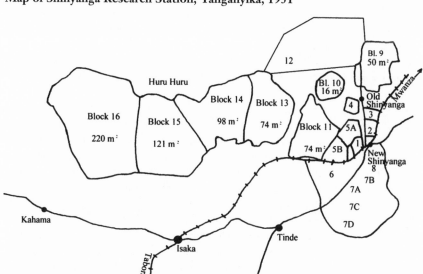

Based on a map in TNA T5/3 215.

TSETSE BARRIERS

The primary focus of research at Shinyanga was on tsetse barriers. The Tsetse Research and Reclamation Department generated plans for various types of tsetse barriers depending on the species of tsetse involved, on environmental conditions, and on different colonial visions of African environment. The colonial idea of clearing barriers beyond which tsetse fly could not pass was based on the understanding that tsetse were advancing along huge territorial fronts into fly-free areas. Colonial scientists in Tanganyika believed that clearing lands of vegetation (which provided tsetse with the shade and cover they preferred) ahead of these fly advances would stop the spread of tsetse. In the next phase of operations the British planned to apply the methods used to clear barriers (burning and hand-cutting vegetation and hand-catching tsetse) in order to eliminate all tsetse from the areas protected behind tsetse barriers. Thus by isolating lands from tsetse advances, it was hoped that strategically placed barriers would render large areas safe for human and animal occupation.

Various barrier-clearing methods defined three major types of landscape central to British perceptions of Tanganyika—each having vastly different implications in terms of environmental impact. When colonial scientists initiated tsetse-control clearing schemes in the early 1920s, they proposed sheer clearing as a standard clearing method. African labor was to clear completely areas of land through controlled burning, cutting down trees and bush, or a combination of the two. Swynnerton initiated controlled burning as tsetse control immediately upon becoming game warden of Tanganyika in 1921.[87] At Shinyanga Swynnerton was interested in the practical application of bush burning, which was an existing component of Sukuma and Zinza agricultural practices that Swynnerton thought colonial regulations could adjust to create fly barriers.

People in southern and eastern Africa often burned vegetation early in the dry season to promote human and cattle access, produce fresh grass growth for grazing, and make it easier to hunt. Some groups organized locally to burn areas, but often farmers and cattle owners set fires independently. In Sukuma and Zinza areas, honey collection was also an important economic activity, and honey collectors set small local fires to smoke out beehives.[88] Swynnerton's criticism of small local burning was that tsetse populations could easily move away from fires and then return to the burned areas as vegetation grew back.[89] His idea was that thorough, well-organized, and controlled large burnings late in the dry season would destroy smaller trees along with dry underbrush, kill tsetse pupae, and deprive tsetse of shade. Late in the dry season, grass, trees, and fallen leaves would be at their most flammable. Fires would be hotter, would draw in more wind, and would more effectively destroy low trees important for tsetse shade.[90]

From 1924 to 1930 tsetse researchers used the 50-square-mile Block 9 as a fire-control area. Tsetse officials depopulated the area and tried to control African access. African employees of the Tsetse Department, referred to by British officials as *fly boys*, regularly surveyed the block along proscribed fly routes to establish fly counts. African fly scouts stopped local farmers and cattle herders from starting fires on their own in the block. Once a year, in September, workers cleared firebreaks and burned the entire block in a massive organized burn. Fly boys would enter any unburned pockets to clear vegetation by cutting and hand-catch the remaining flies. Officials then resumed fly counts to document the effectiveness over time of late burning.[91]

For hand-clearing, African laborers with machetes and axes clear-cut defined areas of all trees and major scrubs. Hand-clearing was usually combined with burning. Controlled burning was not effective over uneven terrain or for limited areas of precise clearing and it was best restricted to a specific time of year. For hand-clearing, in contrast to burning, tsetse control officers could use African labor anytime, anywhere. Hand-clearing combined with burning meant workers dragged cut vegetation into piles, left the piles to dry, and then burnt them, or workers moved through areas after controlled burns and clear-cut any surviving vegetation. To eliminate the difficulty of cutting down and burning live trees, the Tsetse Department advocated ringbarking to kill trees before they were cut and burned and ringbarking combined with the application of tree poisons such as arsenic and saltpeter.[92] Tsetse officers presented vegetation-free, and therefore fly-free, areas as protective barriers for healthy oases of human settlement.

Tsetse scientists also observed that tsetse flies avoided areas with too much vegetation. Researchers conjectured that in such areas fly movement was too hampered, or there was too little food, or flies could not see their food clearly. The logical flip side of controlled late burning, then, was growing vegetation too thick for tsetse habitation. Tsetse scientists called this second type of landscape "densification by fire exclusion." In the 1930s the department placed a 4-square-mile area in Block 4 under protection from fire, extended this experiment to Block 9, and then to a total of 700 square miles by 1938. African labor cleared firebreaks, and fire watchers called out fire brigades to put out accidental fires.[93]

In theory and practice, the idea of densification arose out of depopulated sleeping sickness areas in Uganda at the turn of the century, where scientists believed nature left alone would eventually cleanse itself of sleeping sickness. The American entomologist W. F. Fiske developed the idea of densification in Uganda between 1910 and 1920 from experiments and observations: "Mr. Fiske in Uganda, in converse of Swynnerton, is checking grass fires in certain infested areas to get dense growth of valuable forest trees."[94] In Tanganyika this method proved successful against the savanna tsetse species—G. *morsitans* and G. *swynnertoni*. The problem with densification was that, although densified barriers were maintenance free in theory, in fact fire-fighting and policing of them proved labor-intensive and expensive. Furthermore, such lands were not productive as cultivation areas.[95]

In between these two landscaping extremes (the one of total clearing through fire and cutting, the other of uninterrupted growing), a third kind of controlled landscape was discriminative clearing. Experiments became increasingly sophisticated in connecting how specific kinds of vegetation and combinations of plants and trees promoted the spread of certain tsetse species. The idea was that it was not necessary to cut and burn all vegetation, but that sleeping sickness officials could more effectively use African labor with precise mapping and small surgical interventions. Discriminative clearing would create safe, navigable, latticework environments. Shinyanga researchers carried out experiments in discriminative clearing toward the center of the station in Blocks 1 through 5. From the 1930s through the end of the colonial period, scientists advocated a variety of methods that cleared discriminitively, targeting "vital" vegetation communities.[96] Various methods of discriminative clearing involved the selective destruction of 3 percent to 10 percent of total vegetation cover in various clearing shapes (see figure 4.2).[97] These options, and combinations of these options, allowed tsetse officers flexibility in considering issues of labor availability and costs (discriminative clearing was cheaper than sheer clearing), local topography, erosion control, and conservation.

From the 1920s through the 1950s throughout Tanganyika, African labor cleared hundreds of tsetse barriers in a myriad of sizes and shapes. These ranged from swatches of sheer-cleared land miles long and two-miles wide, to 10-yard-wide clearings along river banks, to discriminative clearings of five-acre stands of a particular kind of bush (see figures 4.2 and 4.3). Colonial scientists debated the minimum width and length of variously shaped clearings necessary to stop the spread of tsetse. The first tsetse-control clearing at Shinyanga was between Kizumbi and Shinyanga on the Tabora-Mwanza Road where Swynnerton directed African labor in clearing a seven-mile-long barrier that fluctuated from 1,000 to 400 yards wide. The barrier cut off a small projection of tsetse-infested bush from the main tsetse area.[98] Tsetse researchers then conducted eradication experiments on the isolated tsetse population in this area. The idea of the dumbbell clearing was in response to researchers conjecturing that tsetse might fly parallel to a fly barrier until its end and then come around the flank. Flies confronted with round clearings at the ends of rectangular clearings would theoretically change direction and veer back towards where they came from.

Figure 4.2
Types of Sleeping Sickness Clearings

Sheer Clearing: Destruction of all plant communities through cutting, poisoning, fire, or various combinations of these three.

Barrier Clearing: Usually sheer. Made in front of fly advance to prevent further country from invasion. 1 to 2 miles wide.

Rod Clearing: Sheer clearing 10 yards wide on each side of rivers.

Discriminative Clearing: Removal of certain plant communities necessary for the survival of tsetse (creating a patchwork effect).

Selective Clearing: Felling certain trees and scrubs throughout an area (creating a thinning effect).

Defense In Depth: Combination of discriminative and selective clearing 5 to 8 miles wide.

Drainage Line: Rod clearing along drainage systems.

Dumbbell Clearing: Sheer clearing rectangle with circular clearing on each end to inhibit tsetse moving around ends of clearing.

Long-Shore Clearing: 200 yards to 2 miles along lakeshores.

Block Clearing: Isolate blocks with sheer cleared perimeters, then discriminative clear, hand-catch and trap to eradicate tsetse.

Road Clearings: 1,000 to 1,500 yards sheer clearing along both sides of a road.

Perimeter Clearing of Great Plain System: 1,000 to 1,760 yards wide through light bush between gall-acacia of plain and true tsetse habitat.

Fire Exclusion (Densification): Prohibit fires to allow vegetation to grow too dense for tsetse infestation.

From *Department of Tsetse Research Report, 1935–1938*, 18, TNA; *Department of Tsetse Survey and Reclamation Annual Report*, 1995, TNA.

Figure 4.3
Aerial View of Sheer Clearing, 1934

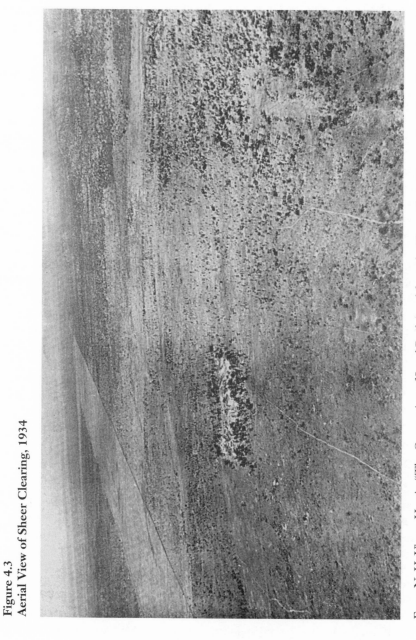

From N. H. Vicars-Harris, "The Occupation of Land Reclaimed from the Tsetse Fly in Tanganyika," *East African Annual*, 1934/35, 2.

Provincial tsetse officers planned clearing schemes according to a compilation of land surveys. Tsetse surveyors, relying on information gathered by local employees, produced fly maps and fly surveys. Fly boys conducted regular fly counting along established routes to map the direction tsetse were moving. Surveys then included a record of tsetse-species movement over time and the boundaries of bush infestation. Tsetse maps included soil types, water sources, elevation, vegetation types, tsetse numbers and species, and human occupation.

Tsetse officials drew up plans of where fly barriers should be cleared to protect the maximum number of people and territory from the spread of tsetse. They supported their proposals with a history of human land use in the area to show the potential value of reclamation and recommended directions for future development. Finally, the clearing proposal estimated labor requirements and clearing costs and presented suggestions for labor and funding sources.[99]

Colonial officials calculated labor in man-days (m/d) according to the body of statistics available about how much labor on average could be accomplished by one adult man in one day, depending on the type of clearing and the type of topography. In late 1923 the Shinyanga District administrator called district chiefs from Shinyanga to meet with Swynnerton. Swynnerton asked for voluntary labor turnouts of adult men with pangas to clear bush for tsetse control. Ten district chiefs sent over 10,000 men to work for the Tsetse Department in 1924. Swynnerton praised local cooperation. He made observations on how best to organize and motivate labor.[100] By 1924 his initial experiments cleared 24 square miles of land. By 1927 in Shinyanga, local African labor had cleared 86 square miles and opened up 200 square miles for settlement and grazing. By the 1930s colonial officials used the working formula that 4,500 man-days were needed per square mile cleared.[101]

CONCLUSION

A combination of broad metropolitan agendas, colonial actions, Africans' interactions with their environments, and environmental changes produced Western images of northwest Tanganyika as desolate wilderness. These images are in marked contrast to images of productivity and luxuriance in Uganda. But similar to the formulation of British sleeping sickness control in Uganda, European perceptions of environments and people, the politics of nature conservation, and the relationship between British colonialism and British science resulted in a particular approach to sleeping sickness eradication. The shift of sleeping sickness research and control to Tanganyika in the early 1920s followed a change in political attention as the epidemic in Uganda abated and tsetse infestation in Tanganyika grew. It was a shift from trypanosomiasis control to tsetse control.

In Tanganyika there was no potentially valuable political and environmental order to protect and reinforce as in Buganda. In the emerging strategies of tsetse prevention in Tanganyika, it was not a question of allying with a centralized African state to resettle people from the margins to an ordered center. The extent of fly infestation resulted in large-scale environmental research and the beginnings of depopulations and resettlement.

Tsetse-control research at Shinyanga under Swynnerton is an important example of how environmental context and environmental politics informed policy. Tsetse-control policy maintained the prominence of colonial natural scientists in entomological and botanical fieldwork and environmental intervention through an alliance with preservationist interests. Sleeping sickness control also began the environmental colonization of remote parts of Tanzanyika by legally and physically dividing environments into development and nondevelopment areas.

NOTES

1. Kjekshus, 162–164.
2. Cooper, 27–28.
3. Buxton, 489.
4. M. Macmillan, *Introducing East Africa* (London, 1952), 259.
5. Thomson, 211, 238, 263.
6. Burton, 7; Kjekshus, 72.
7. Baumann, 59.
8. Weule, 61.
9. Thomson, 211; Kollman, 106; Stanley, 138, 173; Decle, 328; Stuhlmann, *Mit Emin Pasha*, 102.
10. Thomson, 234.
11. Stuhlmann, *Mit Emin Pasha*, 76–77.
12. Baumann, 210.
13. Hore, 60.
14. Ibid., 59; Stanley, 138, 173; Decle; Stuhlmann, *Mit Emin Pasha*.
15. Kollman, 176–178.
16. R. Austin, 180.
17. Audrey Richards, *East African Chiefs* (London, 1960), 207.
18. Cameron, 40.
19. Ibid., 159.
20. Ibid., 239.
21. Ibid., 261.
22. L. Von Brandis, *Deutsche Jagd am Viktoria Nyanza* (Berlin, 1907); Hans Behrends, *Steppenwanderer: aus meinen Pflanzer—und Jagerleben in Ostafrika* (Berlin, 1928); J. Boyd, *My Farm in Lion Country* (London, 1933).
23. Boyd, 13.
24. Pratt, 205.
25. Leroy Vail, *The Creation of Tribalism in Southern Africa* (Berkeley, 1991).

26. Paul Betbeder, "The Kingdom of Buzinza," *Journal of World History* XIII, 4(1971), 736–759.

27. Ibid., 12; Parker Shipton, "Two East African Systems of Land Rights," (unpublished master's thesis, Oxford, 1979), 53.

28. Holmes, 387, 395.

29. Koponen, 245.

30. Shipton, "Two East African Systems," 42.

31. Koponen, 278; Shipton, "Two East African Systems," 57; Malcolm, 27; Hans Cory, *Sukuma Law and Custom* (London, 1953), 7, 126–127.

32. Shipton, "Lineage and Locality," 91–92.

33. Malcolm, 53–54.

34. Shipton, "Lineage and Locality," 63–64.

35. Ford, *African Ecology.*

36. Malcolm, 51; Shipton, "Lineage and Locality," 98.

37. A. Richards, *East African Chiefs*, 198.

38. Ibid., 198.

39. Ibid., 197.

40. Kjekshus, 145–151.

41. Iliffe, 40–55.

42. Ibid., 246.

43. Ibid., 261.

44. W. Rodney, "The Political Economy of Colonial Tanganyika," in M. H. Y. Kaniki, *Tanganyika Under Colonial Rule* (London, 1979), 145.

45. E. A. Brett, *Colonialism and Underdevelopment in East Africa* (New York, 1973); Iliffe, 262.

46. Iliffe, 473–474.

47. Ibid., 70–80; Giblin, 66–68; Koponen.

48. Koponen, 59.

49. Rodney, 134–139.

50. Kjekshus, 157.

51. Ibid., 159.

52. Iliffe, 136–137.

53. Holmes, 400; A. Richards, *East African Chiefs*, 198.

54. Malcolm, 13.

55. Koponen, 172, 356; Stuhlmann, *Mit Emin Pasha*, 108; Iliffe,166.

56. Interview with Alfred Ishaka, Katoro Village, Geita, Tanganyika, September 16, 1994; also see Iliffe, 166.

57. Kjekshus, 161, 126–160; Turshen, 133–139.

58. Baumann, 72.

59. Ibid., 19.

60. Quoted in Kjekshus, 159.

61. Von Lettow-Vorbeck, 11.

62. Kjekshus, 134; Stendel, 659.

63. Maddox, "Gender and Famine," 89.

64. Charles Swynnerton, Memorandum on Game Preservation and Tsetse Control, 1922, TNA 2702.

65. Beck, *A History*, 119.

66. Swynnerton, "An Examination."

67. Ford, *African Ecology*, 201.

68. Mackenzie, *The Empire of Nature*, 237.

69. Mackenzie, "Experts and Amateurs: Tsetse, Nagana and Sleeping Sickness in East and Central Africa," in Mackenzie, *Imperialism and the Natural World*, 199.

70. Mackenzie, *The Empire of Nature*, 214.

71. Mackenzie, "Experts," 204.

72. Nash, *Africa's Bane*, 23.

73. D. and C. Livingston, *Narrative of an Exploration*, 233; D. Livingston, *Missionary Travels*, 365.

74. Stuhlmann, "Notizen," 152.

75. Kjekshus, 54–55.

76. Spreiter, 1908, quoted in Kjekshus, 53.

77. Ralph A. Austin, 196; Swynnerton, *The Tsetse Flies of East Africa*, 8.

78. Ford, *African Ecology*, 221.

79. Ibid., 221–222.

80. Kjekshus, 170–174, based on C. Gillman, *A Population Map of Tanganyika Territory* (Dar es Salaam, 1936).

81. Ford, *African Ecology*, 224–226

82. Hatchell, 60–64.

83. Glasgow, 23, 26.

84. Glasgow, 23; McKelvey, 156.

85. Glasgow, 24.

86. Harrison, 271–293; Glasgow, 28–29.

87. Game Circular No. 734/96, August 7, 1921, reprinted in Glasgow, 31–34.

88. Glover, 603–604.

89. Swynnerton, "An Examination," 325, 382–385.

90. Ibid., 325.

91. McKelvey, 147–148; Glasgow, 24.

92. Swynnerton, "An Examination," 380; Swynnerton, "An Experiment," 326; Bush Clearing Techniques and Costs, Department of Agriculture, 1951, TNA 41470.

93. Glasgow, 24–25.

94. Report from Northern Nigeria, Director of the Imperial Bureau of Entomology, 1921, TNA 2702; also see Ford, *African Ecology*, 13–17, 249–251.

95. Glasgow, 25.

96. Tsetse Department Report for 1955, ZA, Zanzibar.

97. Director Tsetse Research to District Commissioner Musoma, April 24, 1944, TNA 32535; Director Tsetse Research to Provincial Commissioner Lake Province, February 11, 1953, TNA 215 T5/3.

98. Swynnerton, "An Experiment," 320, 323.

99. Tsetse Survey Reports, Northern Province, September 1944, November 1942, TNA 30250.

100. Swynnerton, "An Experiment," 322.

101. Ford, *African Ecology*, 203.

CHAPTER 5

Forced Resettlement in Tanganyika and Uganda, 1935–1960

Beginning in the 1930s British officials began to conceive of sleeping sickness settlements as utopian sites of health and scientific management where all aspects of settlers' lives—economic, political and social—would be reordered and controlled. Sleeping sickness control officers hoped that settlements would be places for the control and modernization of African social structures, production systems, and travel habits. Within the defensive positions of theoretically tsetse-free sleeping sickness settlements, colonial agents imagined reeducating local people to live and produce as modern rational farmers and pastoralists. After reeducation Africans were then to spread back out to reclaim their lands from tsetse in a healthy and orderly manner.

British sleeping sickness policies attempted to control the exact location of and activities of local people, and by doing so, to reorder the relationship between people and nature. The colonial vision of inclusive sleeping sickness control involved thorough surveying, mapping, and intervening in all aspects of human and tsetse activity. Scientists researched relationships between tsetse and specific vegetation communities. The primary approach to tsetse barrier clearing shifted from sheer clearing to more nuanced discriminative clearing.

Planned village resettlement and tsetse barrier brush-clearing became official policy in Tanganyika and Uganda in 1935. To distinguish healthy from unhealthy space, sleeping sickness controls created environmental boundaries. One way for colonial administrations to make boundaries real was to ensure that the lives of Africans changed as they traveled across these borders. Sleeping sickness control scientists identified dangerous African behaviors such as fishing, honey collecting, and hunting that brought people out of settled safe space into fly bush. Colonial officers then enacted controls to limit and regulate these kinds of African production. Moreover, sleeping sickness authorities faced the problem of controlling Africans' movements through fly bush, usually towards centers of wage labor. Because migrant labor moved both within territories and between Uganda, Kenya, Rwanda-Burundi, and Tanganyika, sleeping sickness controls were involved in policing and defining territorial borders. In settlements and at border crossings, tsetse officers mandated medical examinations and pass systems.

An examination of the sleeping sickness control process reveals important links between colonial disease control in Tanganyika and Uganda and environmental, cultural, and economic colonization, showing how colonial science fit into the broader system of British imperialism. Forced resettlement as disease control was an effective colonial mechanism for intervening into the lives of African populations scattered in remote areas. In Tanganyika sleeping sickness control officials based this policy on their perception of African environments as desolate wilderness and on understandings of Africans' relationships to these environments as impermanent and insubstantial. In Uganda, in contrast, the colonial state was more concerned with maintaining peasant productivity.

Local people did not necessarily think colonial agents were lying about sleeping sickness and tsetse. However, most communities were not experiencing a sleeping sickness epidemic. They experienced medical examinations, the British expropriation of land and labor, the loss of investments in homes and farms, and denied access to resources while colonial officials had free access. Local people exchanged information about dispossessions, forced moves, forced labor, medical tests, forced hospitalization, and drug treatments. Colonial sleeping sickness control did not have a good reputation.

Africans used a variety of strategies to resist colonial sleeping sickness resettlement and to adjust sleeping sickness controls to their advantage. They noticed inconsistencies in colonial policy. Forms of resistance to resettlement show not only how remote the colonial logic of sleeping sickness control was to most people, but also the extent to which the human landscapes of fly areas and sleeping sickness settlements were the result of Africans' negotiations with colonial officers and with each other. Local production systems, preferences, and systems of power informed Africans' responses to colonial policy and, therefore, informed colonial practice.

MAPPING AND MOVING

After 1935 colonial mapping and surveying became more detailed and exact. Fly maps identified where medical examinations had found sleeping sickness cases and where people lived, worked, and traveled. The Tsetse Control Department in Tanganyika then targeted areas to be concentrated according to areas overrun by tsetse, according to the direction tsetse was spreading, according to the routes people were travelling, and according to where infected individuals had lived and worked. Surveyors compiled much more detailed information on where people were living and working, road and path systems, political boundaries, topography, vegetation and soil types, water sources, wildlife, crops, markets, and livestock (see figure 5.1).[1]

Tsetse officers determined resettlement sites according to soil fertility, water access, distance from fly fronts, and access to main roads, markets, and political authorities. An important determination was size—how much land each household in sleeping sickness settlements needed and was capable of keeping clear in order to maintain a fly-free environment. Too few people on too much land meant bush growth and tsetse encroachment. Too many people on too little land would result in too few crops to meet people's needs, land conflicts, erosion, soil degradation, and, ultimately, out-migration.

Between 1935 and 1945 scientists and officials developed a standard land-use guide for population density and sustainable agriculture based on projects and studies in Sukumaland. The Sukumaland equation involved changing variables that were both scientifically determined, such as soil fertility and sustainable land use, and statistically determined, such as average family size and livestock population densities:

In one homestead there are on average two tax-payers or a total of seven people with an average of fourteen cattle and ten small stock units (at 5 small stock equaling one stock unit) equals sixteen stock units which produce altogether sixteen tons of manure per annum. This manure is enough to manure eight acres every other year, but the stock require two acres each of pasture, equals thirty two acres plus eight arable equals forty acres equals sixteen homesteads per square mile equals 112 people per square mile, say one hundred.[2]

According to this statistical guide, the minimum population necessary to maintain a fly-free settlement was 1,000 families, with each family receiving from 5 to 15 acres.[3] Colonial scientists adjusted and debated these calculations throughout the colonial period. There was a history of colonial administration establishing, dissolving, and reestablishing settlements as tsetse officials reevaluated settlement sizes and locations according to the most recent scientific conclusions and survey reports.[4]

The moving process became closely supervised. For example, at the Bugomba settlement in Western Province in 1937, first the adult men walked to the new settlement, headmen assigned them plots of land, and they began constructing new homes and clearing and planting new fields. Residents were tax-exempt for the first year to help them through the difficulties of establishing new farms. Colonial officers directed men to plant sweet potatoes and beans the first year, as maize and millet did not grow well the first season in newly cleared fields. Retrieving grain supplies from former farms was vital.[5] Women remained behind to prepare these food stores and other possessions for transportation. After new homes were inhabitable, five one-and-a-half-ton

Figure 5.1
Tsetse Surveys, Tanganyika, 1935–1942

Report on Karagwe Chiefdom, June 15, 1935 TNA 215/660
  1. Gambola Boundaries
  2. Area under Tsetse
  3. Area of uninfected bush
  4. Area grazed
  5. Area under cultivation
  6. Water supplies
  7. Industries
  8. Principle crops
  9. Populations by village of natives
  10. Population by village of cattle, sheep, goats
  11. Number of dukas/market locations
  12. Topographic features

Ikoma Area Sleeping Sickness Survey July 1, 1942 TNA 463
  1. Taxpayers (population)
  2. Communication infrastructures
  3. Area occupied
  4. Topography
  5. Cultivation
  6. Game
  7. Soil
  8. People
  9. Population distribution
  10. Cattle
  11. Timber
  12. Fly
  13. Sleeping sickness cases

Preliminary Survey of Uzinza, B.D. Burtt, Botanist, May, 1937 TNA 25102
  1. Agriculture, population and stock
  2. Natural subdivisions
  3. Geology and soils
  4. Vegetation and fauna
  5. Fly
  6. Potentialities of the country
  7. Actual and suggested development
  8. Fly control measures in place
  9. Appendix I: Zinza tree names
  10. Appendix II: Soil profiles

lorries and a tractor pulling carriage, known as a *road train*, moved people and possessions. Officials told families to cut tracks from the main road to their homesteads and mark them with a flag when they were ready to move. The lorries made an average of three trips daily over a two-month period, with each family transporting an average of one ton of food and possessions.[6] Relocations had proscribed timetables; sleeping sickness guards were empowered to arrest anyone found living or traveling through closed fly areas after a move was complete. After the final moving day, tsetse officials burned homes and other structures on depopulated lands to deter people from returning. People in Katoro and Buselesele villages in western Geita District remembered tsetse control officers as *Bwana Choma* (Mr. Fire).[7]

Once resettlement was complete, some African movement through fly zones between sleeping sickness settlements and in and out of fly areas was necessary to provide labor access to colonial mines and plantations for commerce and to allow for the policing, supplying, and administration of settlements. The colonial state did not wish to eliminate migrant labor from fly areas and could not eliminate interactions between communities. So sleeping sickness officials sought to at least regulate African travel through fly zones. Officials identified essential routes between sleeping sickness settlements and in and out of fly areas. Regulations gazetted these roads as legal and all other roads and paths as illegal.

A settlement officer in 1951, for example, argued that a main road in the Isaka Valley was dangerous—heavily traveled and fly-infested—but that it was vital for commerce and communication, so should not be closed. He proposed that the Tsetse Control Department clear and police the road, and that ordinances close two nearby footpaths in order to force people to use the road exclusively.[8] Labor turnouts cleared legal roads, and African fly guards barricaded, policed, and patrolled both legal and illegal travel routes.[9]

Colonial authorities regulated travel by a system of roadblocks and inspection stations. The Fly Ordinance of 1943 codified a system of "inspection and treatment on request" that sleeping sickness authorities had been using since the 1930s. Fly pickets and cleansing chambers guarded legal routes. Fly pickets, sometimes referred to as "Gland Posts" because of medical exams involving lymph fluid extraction, were two-man inspection stations at the border of fly areas or near major population centers.[10] Fly guards there stopped and checked all motorized vehicles, bicycles, people, and animals using the road, looking for tsetse. Cleansing chambers were deflying buildings in which fly guards usually used smoke to drive flies off vehicles and people, but in the 1950s they also used insecticide sprays.[11] From June 14 to July 31, 1926, fly guards at the picket on the Kware Bridge reported they had inspected 773 motor vehicles, 3,195 pedestrians, and "taken" 30 tsetse, 2 from goats and 1 that had been on a cow.[12] Fly guards at the Kasulu picket in 1954 reported collecting 2,358 flies from 591 vehicles, 467 pedestrians, and 31 bicycles.[13] Tsetse officials used fly-picket counts to determine the spread of tsetse and road use. They regularly shifted the location of posts, closing pickets on less-traveled roads with few tsetse, and picketing roads which surveys identified as heavily used, fly infested, or near recently discovered cases of sleeping sickness. In 1950 there were 40 operational fly pickets in Tanganyika and nine cleansing chambers.[14] Fly guards also inspected for medical passes and sometimes for tax certificates.

Swynnerton experimented with using traffic through pickets as mechanisms of tsetse control. Beginning in 1924 fly guards applied "rat varnish," a mixture of resin and castor oil, to a limited number of cars, bicycles, and people. Swynnerton argued this application both protected people from tsetse bites, as tsetse adhered to the sticky mixture before they could bite and killed the fly. Counting the tsetse stuck to people and vehicles at fly pickets on the other side of fly areas, served as an effective way to monitor fly numbers.[15] For African travelers, fly inspections at fly pickets and inside cleansing chambers were moments of surveillance, physical discomfort, and trespass. The system drove many travelers to avoid legal routes and to move illegally.

PLANNED COMMUNITIES IN TANGANYIKA

> Thus by the apparently simple act of concentration, a population is put
> on the way to prosperity.
>> Tsetse Control Meeting Notes, 1933[16]

There was a transition beginning in the late 1920s to more comprehensively planned resettlement. Charles Swynnerton argued that settlements should eventually be positioned strategically to recolonize tsetse-infested lands, but he was not concerned with the structural organization of settlements. Sleeping sickness officials began to publish plans for standardized resettlement and to implement depopulations and resettlements more consistently in the early 1930s. From the 1920s through the 1950s, the form and implementation of sleeping sickness control depended on the interests and skills of local colonial officials, environmental conditions, and relationships between local people, local elites, and colonial authorities. British colonial sleeping sickness control was never uniform.

In 1935 the tsetse fly committee recommended to the British Parliament that defensive retreat from tsetse was a mistake and that the best form of disease control would be to attack fly and fly brush from concentrated villages of 3,000 to 4,000 people each.[17] This was part of a shift in colonial thinking in the 1930s, formalized in the Colonial Development and Welfare Act of 1940, from indirect rule to more active and interventionist strategies of development and local administration.[18] Any scheme financed in part by the colonial development fund had to show elements of agricultural and economic development.

Colonial authors presented the idea that issues of health could not be seen in isolation from issues of social organization, behavior, and economics. Anne

McClintock links emergent bourgeois British values to the metaphor of clean-liness and the civilizing mission: "monogamy ('clean' sex, which has value), industrial capital ('clean' money, which has value), Christianity ('being washed in the blood of the lamb'), class control ('cleansing the great unwashed') and the imperial civilizing mission ('washing and clothing the savage')."[19] In sleep-ing sickness settlements, officers presented all aspects of development through the lens of health: "With better agriculture, more crops and therefore more money, it will then be possible to start propaganda for better housing, better hygiene and better health in the fullest sense of the word."[20] After 1945 some colonial officials proposed this form of resettlement as a model for the eco-nomic development of the entire rural population of Tanganyika.[21]

Planned-settlement schemes addressed a number of ideological and prac-tical problems for the colonial state at this time. Sleeping sickness control officers were interested in making the idea of concentration as attractive as possible to Africans, other colonial departments (such as the Agriculture De-partment), and British popular opinion. The Tsetse Department sought to mitigate resistance: overt African resistance through migration and illegal set-tlement, criticisms from soil conservationists, and the moral qualms about forced resettlement. A 1943 memorandum from the Tsetse Control and Rec-lamation Department stated, "Prevention of sleeping sickness is only the first and ultimately least of the benefits people derive from compact settlement. Soon all scattered people in Tanganyika will want to be resettled."[22] Colonial scientists argued that the advantages of concentration were not only disease control but also potential for development on all fronts.

In the new settlements, planning was intrusive and comprehensive. Tsetse officers organized local labor to cut 10-foot "traces" demarcating outer pe-rimeters and boundaries between homesteads and between fields and pastures. In Shinyanga District settlement regulations required all farmers to set 3-foot posts at the corner of plots, to dig 6-foot-wide trenches along property lines, and to register their crops and livestock on the property with the local native authority.[23] Settlements were usually geometrically shaped. In theory, as set-tlement populations and abilities to keep land cleared increased, settlement officers would extend boundaries to include new land. Regulations made it illegal for local people to live or herd livestock outside demarcated areas and limited travel in and out of settlements to main roads or paths.

Sleeping sickness control officials planned each settlement, at least on pa-per, to have one medical clinic, one mission, one mission school, and one central market. An agricultural and a veterinary advisor would rationalize pas-toralism and African agriculture. Native authority would set up court and a center of political administration. Settlement officers were to organize the construction of dams and wells to assure dependable water supplies. In the 1950s settlement plans even included plans to improve African recreational opportunities by building soccer fields and tennis courts.[24] Development and order would attract further economic investments and more development. Markets, churches, schools, and clinics would draw people out of homes scattered amid dangerous tsetse brush. Schools and central markets were to serve as vehicles for the dissemination of information about health and tsetse control.

As the colonial administration increasingly emphasized economic development beginning in the 1930s, sleeping sickness settlements became venues for agricultural modernization. In 1933 the territorial director of agriculture argued that people in the Northern and Tanga Provinces were incapable of keeping enough land tsetse free for existing livestock and that they needed to resettle. He wrote, "Tsetse fly may be something of a blessing for the future welfare of the tribe," because it would force people to move into sleeping sickness settlements and shift from pastoralism to mixed farming. His department could then promote plowing, erosion control, and new cash crops.[25]

Settlement planners were challenged in particular by the issue of soil erosion, which became a cause célèbre in British colonial literature in the 1930s. Soil erosion challenged policies of resettlement because colonial scientists blamed it on increased African population and livestock density. The idea of using sleeping sickness settlements as bases for introducing rural people to strategies of soil conservation and sustainable agriculture shifted sleeping sickness control from part of the problem to part of the solution. Sleeping sickness settlements became venues for agricultural micromanagement. Agricultural officers tried to introduce ridging-, crop-, and fallow-rotation systems.

For example, in 1930 sleeping sickness officer G. Maclean suggested multivillage settlements with at least 1,000 people surrounded by a shear clearing one-sixth- to one-quarter-mile wide. Each village would have 10 to 40 families, with 5 acres assigned to each family by local elite. With increasing stock, farms might eventually expand to 8 to 12 acres each. His system of planned crop rotation involved half of the farm always being fallow. On the other half, farmers would divide the land into 6 plots: plots 1, 3, and 4 for cereals, plot 2 for groundnuts, plot 5 for beans, and plot 6 for cotton. Plots would rotate through this crop order for six years, and in the seventh year, farmers would switch the fallow half and the farmed half.[26] In Runzewe settlement in 1946, each settler family had a 10-acre plot. The agricultural officer for the province proposed instructing settlers to plant 3 1/2 acres of sorghum, 1 1/2 acres of mixed beans, maize, and groundnuts, 1/2 acre of cassava, and 1/2 acre of sweet potatoes annually, while leaving 4 acres fallow for sustainable production.[27]

In theory this expanded colonial vision of the sleeping sickness settlements was advantageous for the colonial state and colonial businesses. The provincial commissioner of Lake Province promoted settlements: "Natives get good roads and ports, good access to jobs, developed local markets, and protection from sleeping sickness. The territorial administration gets economic development, easier administration, increased food production, and the advancement of backward people. Mines get sleeping sickness protection, labor, and agricultural produce to feed labor."[28] With concentrations the state had better access to environmentally remote lands and disparate populations: "Small isolated settlements are uneconomic, unenterprising, difficult to administer, and impossible to protect from the ravages of vermin."[29] Settlements with centralized roads, courts, and native authority centers increased the effectiveness of communication and official travel and streamlined tax collection. Accessibility was itself a major problem in the establishment and surveillance of concentrations.

Other colonial departments were interested in expanding their authority by taking roles in these new communities, or at least did not want to be left out. They benefited politically from being part of disease-control efforts. All components of colonial planning in sleeping sickness concentrations involved increased surveillance and instruction of residents. Concentration schemes in the late 1930s included African settlement guards to prevent illegal settlement. The Agriculture Department would post agricultural officers in settlements to promote plowing, haymaking, manuring, systems of fallow, and cash crops.[30] Game scouts would both protect settlers from wildlife incursions and control African hunting.

In spite of these plans, from 1935 through independence, the colonial state did not commit resources in a comprehensive or long-term way to settlements. Sleeping sickness policy makers hoped investments by private institutions and local market forces would generate a momentum for development. For example, they hoped missions in concentrations would help provide medical care and education. In 1934 the colonial state offered mission societies monopoly land grants within settlements "for medical, educational, and religious purposes."[31] Colonial officers considered these three operations interconnected. While some missions and small-scale merchants did move into settlements, there was little of the hoped for outside investment.[32]

Missions, like other private institutions and private investment capital, invested in flourishing settlements and neglected poorer, smaller ones. Mission rivalries within larger concentrations caused the commissioner of the Western Province, F. J. Bagshawe, to establish separate spheres of influence for the White Fathers, Christian Mission Society (CMS), and Neukirchen Mission. He argued that multiple missions in a concentration caused "undesirable opposition and spiritual confusion. The chiefs and people definitely do not desire a second mission."[33] The provincial commissioner set a three-mile barrier between missions. He admonished the missionaries, "Your desire of rival societies to sit on top of and hamper each other is regrettable with two-thirds of inhabited Uha untouched by missionaries. I wish my three-mile limit was ten."[34]

The colonial state gave out mission grants according to the order of applications received. Missions responded by putting in as many applications as they could as quickly as they could. In the first six months of 1934, the White Fathers applied for over 200 mission sites in concentrations. The CMS applied for 100 sites in early 1934 in Kibondo District alone.[35] The applications were far beyond the mission societies' abilities to set up missions (in terms of materials and personnel). They sought to reserve rights to a settlement if it should flourish and grow in the future and to protect themselves from competition. A CMS missionary in Uha referred to competition over settlements with the White Fathers: "We have lost Nyaviumbo. I have heard that they have occupied Uzinza."[36] But these were occupations on paper only.

In 1938 H.M.O. Lester estimated there were 160,000 to 200,000 people in sleeping sickness settlements in Tanganyika. Of them approximately 50,000 did not resettle, but sleeping sickness officers incorporated their existing homesteads into settlements.[37] In 1936 a population map of Tanganyika showed approximately 70 sleeping sickness settlements, most with between 1,000 and 5,000 inhabitants.[38] Through independence, there were always between 50 and 100 sleeping sickness settlements in existence (see figures 5.2, 5.3, 5.4, 5.5).

REGULATING AFRICAN PRODUCTION

As part of the reordering of African production systems in sleeping sickness settlements, officials tried to identify, restrict, and regulate African industries that involved a high risk of exposure to tsetse.[39] Sleeping sickness officers tried to reconstruct the movements of infected individuals to identify where they had been infected. In Runzewe in 1945 and 1946, of 39 traceable cases, case histories showed that tsetse had infected 25 people while they were camping illegally in fly-infested forests, and the remaining 14 had been bitten while traveling to visit friends and relatives.[40] A sleeping sickness survey from northwest Tabora in 1950 listed 72 infected cases broken down by category according to how they were infected: 12 while traveling, 5 fishing, 5 honey hunting, 8 hunting, 8 collecting wood, 3 on roadwork, 5 on railroad work, and the remaining 26 while in settlements.[41] While the majority of cases had been traveling or working outside sleeping sickness settlements, remaining within the boundaries of settlements was not foolproof protection from contracting the disease.

By identifying certain African production systems as dangerous, colonial scientists initiated a process of gathering knowledge in order to apply effective controls. Colonialists studied the African work patterns and technologies involved with honey, wood, and mushroom collecting, iron smelting, fishing, fish curing, transportation, trade, hunting, salt mining, and charcoal production—any productive activity where Africans traveled through tsetse areas.[42] The Tanganyika Territorial Tsetse Committee in 1947 recommended outlawing African hunting parties because hunters resided in bush camps for weeks at a time.[43] Sleeping sickness ordinances in Tanganyika in the 1940s and 1950s prohibited charcoal production in various locations.[44] Settlement officers recorded individuals who kept beehives and how many they kept.[45] Officials recommended that honey collectors be required to keep some hives inside settlements to promote a shift from honey hunting to beekeeping.[46] In the 1950s in Kibondo settlement, officials built two honey-collecting camps to regulate collection, and a beeswax officer worked to promote the marketing

Figure 5.2
Map of Sleeping Sickness Settlements in Northwest Tanganyika

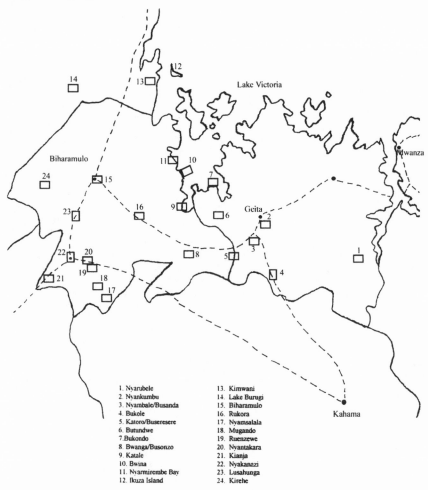

1. Nyarubele	13. Kimwani
2. Nyankumbu	14. Lake Burugi
3. Nyambale/Busanda	15. Biharamulo
4. Bukole	16. Rukora
5. Katoro/Buseresere	17. Nyamsalala
6. Butundwe	18. Mugando
7. Bukondo	19. Ruenzewe
8. Bwanga/Busonzo	20. Nyantakara
9. Katale	21. Kianja
10. Bwina	22. Nyakanazi
11. Nyarmirembe Bay	23. Lusahunga
12. Ikuza Island	24. Kirehe

Based on maps in TNA 10232, 1939.

of wax.[47] Plans for settlements included a forest block within the settlement to give residents controlled access to fuel, building poles, and bark for bee-hives.[48] Sleeping sickness officers characterized fishing camps as dirty and fly infested and they assigned African fish guards to regulate landing conditions.[49]

Colonial sleeping sickness rules required Africans in high-risk occupations in sleeping sickness settlements to register with colonial authorities, receive

Figure 5.3
Map of Sleeping Sickness Settlements, Kibondo, Urambo, and Kasulu Districts

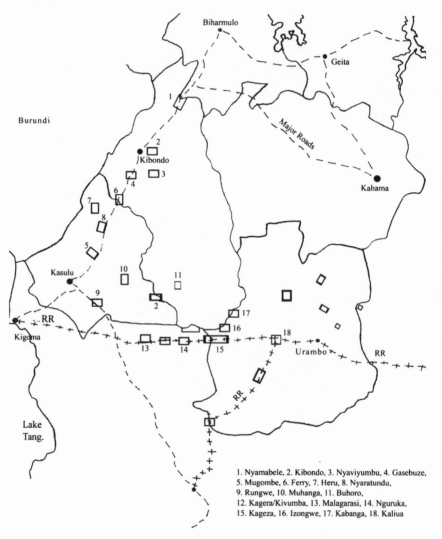

1. Nyamabele, 2. Kibondo, 3. Nyaviyumbu, 4. Gasebuze,
5. Mugombe, 6. Ferry, 7. Heru, 8. Nyaratundu,
9. Rungwe, 10. Muhanga, 11. Buhoro,
12. Kagera/Kivumba, 13. Malagarasi, 14. Nguruka,
15. Kageza, 16. Izongwe, 17. Kabanga, 18. Kaliua

Based on maps in TNA 10232, 1950.

Figure 5.4
Map of Mkalama Sleeping Sickness Settlement, Tanganyika, 1940

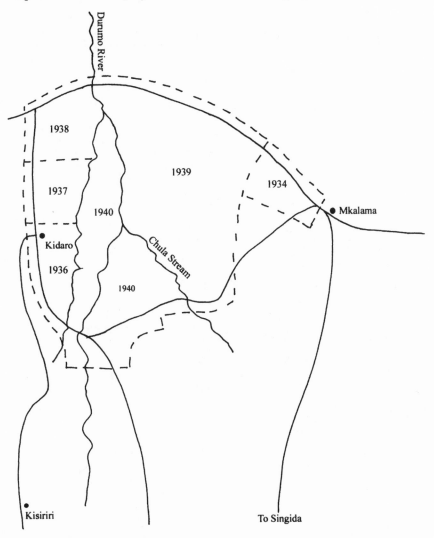

Based on a map in TNA 46 24/5 Vol. 2, 1940.

Figure 5.5
Map of Itimbya Sleeping Sickness Settlement, Tanganyika, 1940

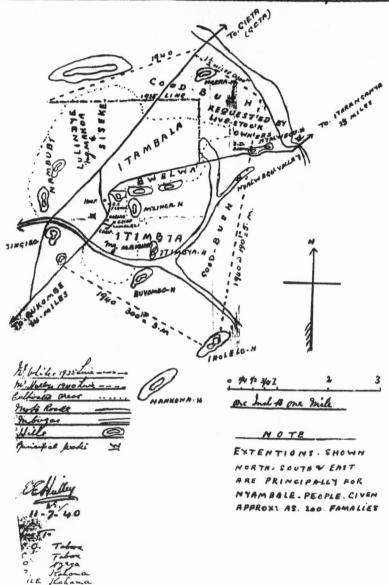

medical examinations, and carry permits and identification. The administration in Tanganyika in the 1940s called for a permit system for honey collectors, hunters, and fishers.[50] Honey collectors and fishers had to carry medical passes to gain access to forests and fishing areas. Passes were good for one month, and settlement guards took blood for blood-slide tests from all people as they returned.[51]

In Uganda and Tanganyika sleeping sickness regulations targeted fishers in particular. Sleeping sickness ordinances in Uganda from 1908, 1928, and 1956 regulated fishing. Canoe owners had to register all canoes annually and paint registration numbers on their bows. All fishers on Lake Victoria had to receive medical examinations in order to receive a fishing permit.[52] In 1923 the medical department examined 5,000 registered fishers biannually.[53] The initial 200 fishers who returned to the Sesse Islands in 1920 had to wear a lead seal around their necks indicating they had passed a sleeping sickness examination.[54] Rules mandated that all Ugandans resettling in sleeping sickness areas from 1920 through 1962 have annual gland exams.[55] In 1937 medical officers examined fishers on Lake Edward and Lake George every three months and treated them with injections of antrypol.[56]

TANZANIAN EXPERIENCES WITH RESETTLEMENT

Responding to an African history of sleeping sickness control, many people moved deeper into illegal fly areas, or waited until resettlement or barrier-clearing labor was complete, then filtered back into their previous home areas. Colonial authorities referred to avoidance and escape from clearing labor and resettlement, and all unregulated migration in fly areas, as desertion. In 1933 of 16,700 families resettled in Kigoma District, settlement officers reported that 18 percent had moved out of the district to other areas, either to other settlements or to non–sleeping sickness control areas, and 16 percent were yet unaccounted for.[57] In Bukoba in 1935, 24 percent of the families concentrated from Nyabionza and Nyaishozi areas did not show up in the designated resettlement area.[58] In 1943 the provincial commissioner of Lake Province wrote that a 15 percent desertion rate from settlements was normal.[59]

Africans were always moving in and out of settlements illegally to work and travel in fly zones. They ignored and circumvented pass systems, sneaking in and out or claiming they had lost their passes. People resented the economic and social restrictions in settlements and close colonial supervision: "The place would be ruled by whites. There were rules about walking to gather wood and water, and visiting people to do business or just visiting family. No one can make those kinds of rules. People didn't listen to chiefs trying to enforce them."[60] Settlement guards arrested and fined people for illegal hunting, honey and wood collection, and for being in illegal areas.

Local responses were not simply resistance to colonial coercion, but involved local power relationships. For example, there was a generational and gendered element to out-migration as a response to the threat of resettlement. In Katoro, Salvatory Kalema spoke of young men taking orders to relocate as an opportunity to migrate on their own: "Older people with families could do nothing, but many younger men, even some with wives and young children, would leave."[61] Men in Biharamulo remembered, in contrast, that families with labor and material investments in farm land and buildings often refused to move: "Sometimes a man's father had been born on the same land, and a family had buildings and businesses and animals. To force people to leave was theft."[62]

Resettlement actions involved colonial officers as variables in local political contexts. Local elite negotiated from their position between the colonial state and local labor. They weighed the advantages of cooperating with the state, and therefore having the state reinforce their authority from above, with alienating local constituencies and having their authority undermined from below. There were potential advantages to having colonial-state backing and authority over basically captive populations in settlements. Settlements with fertile soils, good water and fishing sources, or a good commercial location in relation to other population centers, such as Ulanya and Biharamulo, flourished and expanded. Elite in successful settlements accumulated wealth and power, while elite in failing settlements, or those who failed to convince their constituency to resettle, lost people to out-migration.

In a detailed example of the Buyombe resettlement in 1934–35, the first village meeting, or *baraza*, when a tsetse surveyor explained the policy of settlement, was lively and well attended. Such meetings were the basis of British justifications of sleeping sickness settlements as voluntary. At the meeting, after a presentation on tsetse and resettlement by the surveyor, Charles Macquarie, local residents asked a number of questions then deliberated among themselves for two hours. Chief Edward Ludamila informed Macquarie that everyone had agreed on an area for relocation to the north. This was not an area of choice for Macquarie, who then told the meeting why his choice was superior to theirs. According to Lamb's report, after further discussion "it was decided that the headmen and elders should accompany Mr. Macquarie to the part of the district particularly recommended by him." Soon after this, Lamb received a letter from the local elite saying they agreed on Macquarie's site choice, but cautioned the district officer about the limitations of their power in this instance: "They reminded me, however, of the fact that their people had selected Nyambale and asked that they should not be made a laughing stock if their villagers refused to follow their advice and carried out their threats to move to other chiefdoms."[63]

Macquarie's next trip to the new settlement site was to show residents the land he and the local elite had agreed upon. In a letter from some of the inhabitants of Buyombe to the district officer, the authors write that when Macquarie told them this was the land chosen for their resettlement, "We did not do anything, but kept silent, for his words made it clear that it was a matter of government compulsion to move us. We were afraid at the time to make any answer to the words he explained to us."[64] Processes of explanation and choice in these meetings were defined by power relationships, as Bazage Kanumi in Biharamulo responded to my question about whether resettlement was voluntary: "Every person always has a choice. But in deciding what to do, people thought about the consequences of opposing the head of the family, chief or white person."[65] According to Kanumi, local Africans placed settlement officers as part of a continuum of power.

In the letter from the citizens of Butundwe to the district commissioner, they reported that the local elite had not shown up for the second tour with Macquarie. Villagers took this as a sign that they had been cut out of site selection negotiations. In local elites' concerns about not being obeyed, and in not touring the land with Macquarie and local people, they were responding to the vulnerability of their position between colonial and local interests. Elite power depended on both these groups, and in this case chiefs were negotiating their positions by playing both sides.

There was also competition between chiefs over fertile areas and relocated people. In 1957 Mwami Kandege wrote the district commissioner (DC) at Mpanda that a neighboring chief was setting up new illegal boundaries, rejecting all the old "marks and lines which the survey did . . . claiming that he knew better and saying there were two lines instead of one." Kandege called on the DC to intervene and issued a direct threat: "Now we are confused, and would rather go back to the forest than stay here unpeacefully."[66] Sleeping sickness settlement guidelines recommended that officers require chiefs to accompany them when cutting traces, so chiefs could not "plead ignorance about illegal territories."[67] Mrisho Selemani Migila offered the Sleeping Sickness Control Department 1,000 Tanganyika shillings to help pay for the relocation of people into his territory.[68] Rival chiefs contested the extensions of settlements. In some cases chiefs balked at relocations that would settle their former subjects on land claimed by another chief. In Ukonongo, the DC assured chiefs that if they cooperated with relocation, chiefs would receive the taxes of former subjects, no matter where subjects decided to settle.[69]

Local people also used desertion and refusal as a threat in negotiating resettlement. In Buyombe, people agreed to move if officials granted them their first site choice in relocation. In other settlement actions, people negotiated for more land in the settlement site or to be allowed to remain where they were in return for clearing the area of tsetse brush. They complained new areas were infertile or too near hostile neighbors.[70] People argued that if not the state then strangers might eventually claim the farms they were now abandoning.[71] Fishers feared they would lose access to good fishing waters. Groups of Warongo, who specialized in iron smelting, were particularly resistant to relocation away from iron ore deposits and fuel sources. They argued for their own independent settlements where they could access ore, balked at resettlement deadlines, and threatened to flee.[72]

According to colonial ratios of the minimum number of farmers necessary to keep a settlement cleared, excessive out-migration made settlements unsustainable. Settlement officers closed and reconstituted settlements, moving groups of people around repeatedly. Chief Selemani Ikamazya of Ussangi in Western Province complained that a sleeping sickness officer had relocated him in 1938, another official had allowed him to return to his original lands in 1948, and then in 1950 granted an exemption from moving yet again. Finally a third officer ordered him to relocate in 1953: "Since 1938 the government has been shifting people and ever since I have never rested."[73] Cycles of resettlement, out-migration, and re-resettlement further reinforced local people's beliefs about sleeping sickness control as political and ad hoc.

Tsetse-control officials recognized the limits of their power in the face of popular resistance to resettlement. Settlements flourished or floundered according to patterns of migration outside of colonial control. In 1939 a tsetse surveyor from Geita advised, "The people just move if 'crossed,' so try to upset them as little as possible at barazas."[74] The colonial state offered villagers relocation incentives of tax exemption, free transportation, seed, and food and made threats of imprisonment and fines. Beginning in the 1930s sleeping sickness officials held out the promises of the planned settlement. They offered chiefs cash incentives to support relocation and threatened to cut off official salaries if chiefs didn't cooperate.[75]

Sleeping sickness officials sometimes adjusted the location of settlements according to popular resistance. In 1928 tsetse-control officers moved the people of Isanga to Ihapula, except for 40 families of ironworkers who refused to move. Officials allowed them to remain at Isanga in an independent settlement. By 1936 enough people had illegally moved back to Isanga such that it was a larger settlement than Ihapula. Sleeping sickness officials decided to resettle people back to Isanga out of Ihapula. The people remaining in Ihapula "refused point blank to move to Isanga." Officials then tried instead to make an entirely new settlement for both groups next to the former settlement at Ihapula. This time the ironworkers refused, "putting every obstacle in the way of the Government."[76]

In another example, Charles Macquarie reported in 1939 that Mlandu Luswabi, already arrested once for illegal settlement, had founded an illegal settlement where "he called himself chief, and was attracting other illegal residents to the Kagembi forest area." Macquarie admitted that there would be advantages to legalizing the settlement, although he opposed rewarding Luswabi's criminal actions.[77]

For their part, tsetse-control officers sometimes extended settlements to integrate nearby squatters. Illegal settlement around the outskirts of settlements was common. Sleeping sickness officials were faced with a choice between promoting settlement growth, even if new settlement was on illegal land, or of strictly enforcing regulations and driving people off nearby settlements. In Busonzo, sleeping sickness officials extended settlement boundaries to include squatters.[78] In Ulanga settlement in 1951, settlement officers legalized the practice of living inside the settlement and farming outside. In this "leap-frog" system, when settlement residents had thoroughly cleared and cultivated the most recent perimeter, officials extended the residential boundary to include these farmlands, thus creating a new farming frontier.[79]

The unmet promises of planned settlements further informed African relationships to sleeping sickness control and the colonial state. The fact that health care is currently inaccessible to my informants in Geita District proved to them that resettlements were never really about disease control. They recalled the colonial promise of medical aid. Some sleeping sickness settlements were staffed by an African dresser in a clinic, so were, thereby, places where better health care became available. But in Katoro, for example, the clinic was closed during World War II, and other colonial promises of aid never materialized: "The English had no plans of bringing development here. They paid low wages or just gave us food, but then we had to pay taxes. We were brought together by the road, which was the only positive result."[80] According to Rutekelayo Ifunza from Katoro, resettlement was primarily a mechanism for the British to increase the number of taxpayers. Here again, he gives no credibility to tsetse control as improving local health.

Local people sometimes resisted resettlement through the logic of the colonial system and through ambiguities within colonial ideology. Some African appeals against resettlement, for example, argued the people did not reject the idea of resettlement itself, but the use of force. The people of Buyombe wrote, "We are agreeable and willing to do as others have done, but—and this is our last word—we want only the place we chose [to be resettled in]. We have no other difficulty with which to trouble the Government, except of compulsion."[81] As villagers presented themselves as agreeable to resettlement, colonial officials could not accuse them of being unscientific and irrational. The emphasis on the issue of compulsion here, a concern local people repeated in other resettlement documents as well, indicates an African awareness that the British were concerned with the issue of free choice in colonial rule. Villagers drew on the Western discourse of liberty, portraying themselves as justly resistant to tyranny. Requests voiced in this way placed the British in the position of tyrants if they refused.

The letter from the residents of Buyombe balanced an appeal to liberty at the beginning with an appeal to the paternalism of colonial rule at the end: "We have no alternative but to trust that they will be patient with their children—for a crying child must be given what he wants, otherwise he continues to cry." The strategy of the letter's authors may have been to position themselves as children to provoke sympathy and understanding.

A further local strategy was to draw on previous colonial decisions to challenge current ones. During settlement surveys in the 1940s and 1950s, Tsetse Department officers received much of their information on existing settlement boundaries from residents. These settlers often relied on the authority of previous tsetse officials to justify their claims. The tsetse surveyor C. Macquarie wrote, "There are bush villages on the paths to Nyonga and Kiwere. The Wanangwa say these were left with Dr. Maclean's approval." And in the same report he wrote, "One of the chief's counselors asserted that the late Meta petitioned Dr. Maclean for permission to make these boundaries, and that he gave it."[82] In 1953 in an appeal to the district commissioner of Tabora not to be relocated, Selemani Ikapazya wrote that the DC had given him permission to stay.[83] In these cases local people used the authority of the colonial state to back up their claims. By presenting current arrangements as sanctioned by sleeping sickness officers from the past, settlers put current officials in the position where questioning Africans' claims would undermine officials' own authority. A surveyor explained in 1942, "Contradicting the statements of the chiefs would have undermined their and my authority, as it would have brought into question the wisdom of decisions by officers in the past. If I do not recognize a surveyor's work, why should they."[84]

In 1951 four Luo men in Geita used the colonial legal system to win economic compensation and time. They began writing letters to colonial officials challenging their eviction. The four were among those whom sleeping sickness officials were evicting from the Nyarugusu settlement, comprising 33 homesteads located between the Ralph and Mawe Meru mines in Geita. Most sleeping sickness policy refugees were small-scale farmers with minimal experiences with the colonial state. Gold mining in Lake Province, however, concentrated cash-economy labor and drew African entrepreneurs from Uganda, Kenya, and Bukoba to new market centers.

According to letters written by the four Luo men, and a report by the area chief, Nyarugusu was initially settled in the mid-1940s, and mine management encouraged agricultural production, stores, and hotels to attract a stable workforce. A village headman was appointed by the Bukoli chief, thus further condoning settlement.[85] A district officer conducting a fly survey of the area in May 1951 reported the illegal settlement and warned inhabitants they would have to relocate. On August 1 the DC ordered people out by September 30. Initially, most families began to prepare to move either to existing settlement areas or onto mine lands. Six families of workers moved onto Ralph's mine land.[86]

With the legal challenge by the four Luo men, however, people stopped moving. The September 30 deadline expired, the local native court issued summonses, and the Nyarugusu settlers ignored these as well.[87] Playing components of the system off one another, the four men had sent copies of the initial September 14 letter to the local DC, the director of medical services, and the chief secretary. As colonial officials recognized that both villagers and other colonial officials were aware of the challenge (i.e., it became an official matter), they postponed the eviction. On September 27 the provincial commissioner wrote to the DC, "I assume that no notices of any sort have yet been served by you as the whole issue is still under consideration."[88]

The initial September 14 letter played on a number of ambiguities in colonial policy and on ideological weak points, revealing the political acumen of the "bush lawyers":

This eviction has considerably undermined our present general outlook. We have lived in this area for a considerable period and we have established our homes ever since. It is about seven years now we are in occupation of this land. It is alleged that, we are told to move away from this land because of tsetse flies and wonderful enough we find that our neighbors, like Geita Gold Mining and Co. are not evicted. We have lived with our animals very happily and we have not seen any case of illness occurring from us; and deaths are from natural causes.

Again referring to the Geita Gold mining which . . . is near our residences and there has been nothing said to them, yet we find Europeans, Asians, and Africans living at this place without troubles of contracting sleeping sickness. We have reasons to believe that this movement has been brought about by the DC who is asking us to leave our homes and Shambas unnecessarily; for he thinks we are gaining much.

Funny enough, we just wondered whether these tsetse could distinguish the African blood and that of non-African; whether the African blood was sweetest compared with other bloods. We suspect that the present moves have been caused by our present DC, Mr. Nickol, as there was no such action taken until he took over. . . . This, indeed, has had a very severe effect on our part for some of us possess shops and other cattle wealth. . . .

We shall still be most grateful to you if you could get us a medicine that will stop ndorobos from biting Africans and hence stop our moving way.[89]

The men made charges of racism both in terms of officials' not evicting the mining operations and the DC's resenting African prosperity. The authors brought science to bear with evidence of human and animal longevity in the area and by claiming they were willing to take drug treatments.

The men hired Patel and Patel Advocates in Mwanza to represent them. The lawyers argued that because a village headman existed, and the claimants had paid the headman customary land dues, they were legally "lessees," and at least deserved compensation for lost properties. The DC rejected this claim, stating that only alienated land could be legally leased from the state and that native authorities determined land rights to all other lands. Local native authorities denied giving the four men land rights. But Nickol acknowledged that because the administration had seemingly condoned an illegal settlement for several years (by dint of ignoring it), some compensation was justified.[90]

The controversy prompted follow-up surveys by the DC and a medical officer. On November 6 the provincial commissioner replied to the four Luo men (Edward, Vincent, Orochi, and Jolam) that Nyarugusu was a sleeping sickness risk and would be evacuated.[91] Internal correspondences condemned Nyarugusu as "a hot-bed of crime," where little cultivation was being done, but where income was generated by the "dubious activities of thieves, prostitutes, moshi-distillers and bhang growers."[92] Officials labeled the Luo men foreign troublemakers whose "verbose claims were completely unfounded" and who would do well to exercise "a little responsibility and self-control."[93]

As the DC had promised compensation, authorities in late 1952 offered each of the four claimants 700 shillings for their lost property. Three of the men picked up the compensation money, but Vincent Olutoch refused. He remained at the illegal settlement and, in a letter from May 1953, reiterated his claims against the DC and the mining company. He argued the DC had assessed his household at 14 percent of its real worth, which he put at 8,000 shillings. Olutoch listed the value of nine years of bush clearing, farming expenses, house-building supplies and labor, and the "troubles and disturbance created since the removal scheme was brought into existence."[94]

The next month (June 1953) sleeping sickness guards arrested Olutoch and burned the dwellings in Nyarugusu. The Geita District court jailed him briefly for refusing resettlement and again offered him 700 shillings compensation. Olutoch refused, returned to Kenya, and died in Kisumu in 1954. In 1956 his brother in Kisumu petitioned the Geita District government for the 700 shillings. The DC rejected the request and wrote to the provincial commissioner, "It was thought that all our wasted time and trouble were finally at an end with his death, but evidently his soul still goes marching on."[95] The provincial commissioner paid Olutoch's brother in May 1956 after a crown council advised the district administer to avoid resuscitating the "disrepute of the case."[96]

In the Nyarugusu example, as with African uses of the rhetoric of paternalism and liberty, people targeted for resettlement resisted by using contradictions within the colonial system. As Africans were using the logic and processes of the colonial state to support their claims, colonial officials could not reject their arguments out of hand without undermining the legitimacy of colonial authority itself.

RESETTLEMENT IN UGANDA

Officially the colonial state in Uganda reopened sleeping sickness areas in fits and starts according to a combination of variables: official sleeping sickness reports of fly counts in the proposed area; official reports of the number of sleeping sickness cases in surrounding areas and among work parties in the closed area or among squatters; the reported effectiveness of native labor parties at keeping designated roads and beach landings cleared of bush; African initiatives in the form of formal petitions; de facto land and resource use (squatting and poaching); and the conditions to which Ugandans were willing to agree. A chief from Sigulu Island explained that his parents had made a special agreement with a colonial sleeping sickness officer in the 1950s; they could return alone to their lands for a six-month test period, but only after fly boys trapped flies from their land, and the couple allowed themselves to be bitten by these flies. If his parents were still alive and healthy after the six months (which they were), the officer agreed to open the area to resettlement.[97]

These variables tended to trigger one another in a variety of orders: for example, an African petition bringing on a survey trip, or a survey of reported squatters bringing on petitions. One further colonial consideration was the estimated number of people who wanted to move back into depopulated areas. Sleeping sickness authorities feared allowing large groups back because they feared high population densities would reignite an epidemic. In contrast, they feared small groups returning would not be able to keep up necessary clearing duties. Officials denied resettlement for both reasons.[98]

Africans applied pressures at various political levels for resettlement. In Busoga, where there were no formal colonial land agreements as in Buganda, one level of land politics took the form of written petitions from former residents and requests from chiefs.[99] At a more spontaneous and popular level, dislocated Ugandans wrote letters or asked passing colonial officers when they could return to their lands. A letter from five former Bomba Island residents to the colonial district officer in 1926 asked for permission to return to the island, explaining, "People from islands do not like to be in some part of the country where they were not born."[100] Petitions that reached district officers often led to Tsetse Department investigations.

There were both internal and external politics to African petitions. Ownership was ambiguous due to emptied islands and the fact that lands in Busoga and Buvuma were not governed by formal colonial land agreements. A petition at the right time for the right place might allow a chief to move in on valuable fishing grounds or former market areas. A Soga chief complained that the government had given his island to a Ganda chief while he himself, the rightful owner, had repeatedly asked for access.[101] The territorial administration in Entebbe decided between the rival claims of Busoga Chief Luba and Buvuma Chief Mbubi over islands in the Buvuma Island group. First the government divided the disputed islands equally, giving each chief eight islands. Then the government placed all the islands under Luba's jurisdiction, then finally under Mbubi's.[102]

The history of sleeping sickness control on Buvuma Island is an illustrative case study of the influence of local actions on colonial policies. The colonial state legally depopulated the Buvuma Island group in 1909. Sleeping sickness officials reopened the main island to resettlement in 1921. Buvuma chiefs maintained a government extra-territoriality since 1910, but returned in 1921 with many fewer people than before the depopulation.[103] Settlers could legally settle anywhere on the island, although there were sleeping sickness guards to promote landing clearings and dense settlement. Many islanders returned again to the mainland during an epidemic in the northern part of the island from 1943 to 1944, but sleeping sickness officers didn't close the island. This was partially due to limited colonial resources and chiefs' resistance. Instead, from 1947 to 1948, regulations mandated quarterly injections of antrypol for all inhabitants. Bavuma resented and avoided the injections and sleeping sickness officials discontinued them. After discontinuing the shots though, officials closed the northern part of the island and concentrated people in the south. In 1950 blood slides revealed 50 cases of sleeping sickness among islanders, and sleeping sickness officials advised another complete depopulation. Again, chiefs strongly opposed the idea and in 1951 sleeping sickness rules for Bavuma made evacuation voluntary, quarantined remaining islanders to the island, and mandated blood exams. Only 10 percent of the total island population emigrated to the mainland. Sleeping sickness guards could not enforce the quarantine as people moved to and from the island by canoe and traveled through the northern closed area. Again in 1952, sleeping sickness officials advised a complete depopulation of the island.[104] However, the state continued to be unwilling to risk the political fallout and never officially supported the depopulation of Buvuma again.

Through the 1940s "legal" sleeping sickness resettlement simply meant sleeping sickness regulations opened areas to habitation, thus reestablishing a natural environment by reintroducing healthy humans with a few sanitary improvements to "restock it with healthy natives."[105] The state provided islanders with transport to give them time to rebuild their destroyed canoe fleets. Sleeping sickness officials mandated that markets had to be in official clearings in reopened areas and that farming had to take place beyond a certain minimum distance from the lakeshore. But there was little colonial enforcement of these regulations. Overall, officials made few efforts to restructure human behavior and environment on the Lake Victoria islands. Colonial officers in Entebbe and Jinja looked out across the lake to again see canoes appearing and disappearing according to their own time and season.

Sleeping sickness control policy changed again after World War II. The colonial state took a more direct role in tsetse control and resettlement, partially for the reasons David Anderson presented of British concerns about global erosion and African food production invigorating colonial intervention in the 1930s, and partially in response to a sleeping sickness epidemic that broke out in southern Busoga from 1940 to 1942. In light of the 1940 epidemic, and subsequent small outbreaks through 1963, colonial scientists depicted prewar patterns of resettlement as haphazard and therefore dangerous. They argued that the lack of colonial settlement control was to blame for more recent epidemics and that epidemics would continue to occur without strict sleeping sickness control interventions and enforcement.[106]

Sleeping sickness authorities in Uganda modeled new control initiatives after Tanganyikan schemes. They targeted southern Busoga as a pilot settlement project where new methods would be tested then applied to the rest of Uganda.[107] The 1948 development plan proposed establishing a 50-yard "defense line" along 22 miles of the main Jinja-Kenya road and opening the 50 yards to the north of this cleared barrier for settlement.[108] The colonial state did not commit substantial resources to the plan, and African farmers were not attracted to the overgrown plots. In 1956 sleeping sickness officials began a revised development scheme in the same area. Initially, organized teams of African labor cleared and measured plots along the main east-west road according to a "linear plan, clearing 300 foot strips on either side of the road with 150 foot minimum plot frontage."[109] Ugandans already regularly traveled the road, so the plan sought to define and control existing behavior. Clearing teams were mobile, relatively self-reliant, and included diggers, cooks, hunters (for food procurement), and surveyors.[110] Local chiefs, newly resettled on their old lands, distributed 10-acre plots to settlers in return for *enkoko* (a tenant's one-time-only payment for land to the chief). Colonial settlement planners designated special plots for fishing people, water access points, trading centers, medical clinics, and areas for subsidiary industries such as sand digging, timber, and brick making. They considered a poll-tax exemption for immigrants. Medical officers tested and registered each new resident. Settlement officers would register and control all fishermen and fishing canoes. The settlement formula (like the Sukumaland equation) considered population density relative to labor needed to maintain clearing. Officials demarcated cleared public roads and paths.[111] As in Tanganyikan settlements, reeducation and ordered living were to provide a basis for the eventual healthy recolonization of tsetse-infested Ugandan shores and islands.

In the southern Busoga resettlement project in Uganda, J. T. Fleming, the resettlement officer, faced immediate challenges from local leaders and from a nascent nationalist political organization, the Uganda National Congress (UNC). Four claimant chiefs, including one who had already resettled as a common fisherman on Saguttu Island, came forward. All four opposed the plan for various reasons. A state had recently proposed a land tenure plan for open-land sales in Busoga. Fleming reported that UNC agitators had preceded him into the area and organized chiefs' resistance to the plan.[112] The UNC won the support of local hereditary chiefs who did not receive salaries (and therefore recognition) from the state. Chiefs supported the UNC because chiefs were concerned that the colonial government was moving to alienate their former lands permanently.[113] Ironically, the petty-bourgeois-based UNC opposed resettlement because, in fact, elected parish committees chaired by parish chiefs would be allocating lands, collecting fees, and administering the new settlers.[114] Locally elected committees would exclude urban-based petty bourgeois influences. Fleming was frustrated that chiefs would ally with their political enemies (the UNC) against their own better interests (as he saw them). He spent much of 1956 lobbying the chiefs to support resettlement. He argued that they would still have local administrative control of their lands and that a chief in nearby Bunya had made 5,000 shillings in March alone on plot fees in a newly resettled area.[115]

But the chiefs rightfully recognized the plan as an erosion of their former powers, and internal competition increased their concerns with the plan. Chiefs were concerned that settlers would first fill up one chief's area of plots, leaving other chiefs at a disadvantage. While some farmers and fishers might be loyal to an area, waiting for their own former lands to reopen, they had no particular loyalty to former chiefs, and the resettling population was a new ethnic mixture of Ganda, Gisu, and Soga. One strategy chiefs adopted to protect their future interests was to waylay potential settlers on route and settle them illegally on land not yet cleared. Chiefs settled these squatters on land that would eventually fall within their respective jurisdictions, thus guaranteeing future revenue.[116]

In 1956 Fleming was impatient to move the project along to "get people on land before it reverts to bush" and to keep ahead of unofficial settlement in closed areas.[117] Illegal fishing and squatting abounded. Fishers operating illegally in fly zones shifted to marketing dry fish so they could leave their catch on drying racks at landings. They would then return at night to collect the processed product and claim at market that the dried fish was imported from a legal fishery.[118] Fleming conducted occasional raids, in February 1957 confiscating seven bicycles, 24 nets, and tools from a dozen fishing poachers near Bugoto landing. It was easy for him to catch poachers: "Just walk down to the lake, [but] I dislike harrying these harmless people fulfilling a normally desirable task. . . . we need to get the port open."[119] Fleming negotiated with illegal settlers by moving boundaries to legalize some squatters while evicting others at chiefs' expense (to deter the strategy of waylaying immigrants).[120] In 1959 Fleming revised the initial linear plan to a block plan to incorporate illegal settlement. Two east-west roads were created, one mile apart, with north-south crossroads also one mile apart. This demarcated square-mile blocks. The scheme was to move settlers block by block onto geometrically cleared grids (see figure 5.6). Once 64 families had settled the plots in Block 10, for example, Fleming would open Block 11 for resettlement. But settlers sought only plots fronting roads or landings, while ignoring others. Chiefs continued to fear their blocks might never be settled. Feelings of hostility to the plan and pressures for unified resistance were such that the first chief to give in to Fleming's pleas and support resettlement, Chief Basiibe, fled his new administrative holdings to escape the retribution of his peers. Local chiefs never ceased to involve themselves in the application of settlement plans by resisting, and then negotiating, compromises to their perceived benefit.

Fish and charcoal continued to be important cash sources for Ugandans, and this added to trespassing in closed areas. Considering the extent of lakeshore and islands in sleeping sickness areas, sleeping sickness officers never had the resources necessary (manpower and boats) to police infected areas.

Figure 5.6
Map of Kityerera Resettlement, Uganda, 1960

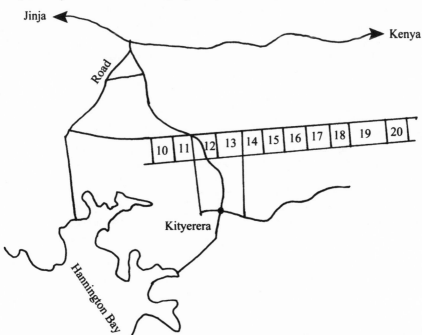

Based on a map in D. H. H. Robertson, "Human Trypanosomiasis in South-East Uganda," *Bulletin of the WHO* 28(1963), 636.

The map compiled by Robertson from officers' reports and aerial surveys between 1958 and 1960 located over 70 illegal fishing camps in Busoga. Only large camps were visible from the air. The illegal camps located on the map near the police harbor at Dagusi Island are indicative of how ineffective sleeping sickness regulations were (see figure 5.7).[121]

Although the colonial state continued to offer incentives—moving immigrants to planned villages at government expense, supplying free tools and seeds, tax exemption, and free iron roofing sheets—farmers and fishers pursued their own land tenure systems and shied away from clearing what was now forest and neglected roads. At the end of 1957 only 54 families had settled in the Kityerera scheme and only 68 fishers had registered.[122] Colonial officials despaired at the disregard of government regulations and resettlement orders. In 1961 the Ugandan colonial state declared the Kityerera resettlement scheme a failure and withdrew all government funds.[123]

Ugandans saw some opportunities in planned settlements. Chiefs with the power to distribute developed farm plots in the Kityerera scheme raised the price of *enkoko* for settlers from 20 shillings to over 500 shillings.[124] Some individuals perceived political authority as up for grabs to the most convincing (and most cooperative) claimant. From May to July 1963, Brighton O., writing from Mombasa, corresponded with the DC in Jinja about resettlement and political authority on Sigulu Island. He employed a number of strategies to advance his bid as chief—that he was an original inhabitant of the island, that he understood ideas of development and hygiene, and that he would be a just and strict tax collector:

There is no reason why I should not be allowed to live in my own island which is Sigulu Island near Busoga District. Since in 1956 we tried all our level best if it could be possible to be allowed to return to our own island, because our grandfathers were the owners of the island and the Ugandan government does not agree to our return. . . . All the members of this island do not agree to pay the personal tax to be taken by the Ugandan government so they find it better to pay the personal tax and go to the Kenyan government. Chiefs are being sent from other places and go there to arrest and treat them unfairly. . . . I will be grateful if you choose the particular

Figure 5.7
Map of Lake Victoria Fishing Camps, Busoga, 1958

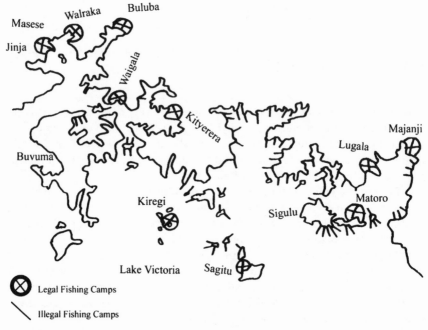

Based on a map in D. H. H. Robertson, "Human Trypanosomiasis in South-East Uganda," *Bulletin of the WHO* 28(1963), 628.

chief for the island. Regards to my qualifications, I was employed by the Royal East African Navy and I worked under the department for ten years and three and one half months. . . . The people need hospital, school and a doctor for animals. They are very ignorant and not up to modern standards, needing a chief who understands their needs.[125]

The sleeping sickness commission had allowed a trial fishing camp and controlled settlement on the island several years before, and the DC informed Brighton the government was allowing no further settlement there at that time for health reasons. Brighton was out of whatever new political loop had emerged since his eviction. He persisted, however, to the point that the DC toured the island in July and found Brighton's claims "exaggerated." A final official letter informed Brighton that his "allegations appear based on emotion and personal recognition and gain. . . . further correspondence if required should be taken up with the Sleeping Sickness authorities, but not with this office."[126]

Other Ugandans benefited from the depopulation and repopulation of lands and viewed sleeping sickness control accordingly. Alexander Salongo Mugenyi claims he bought Mpuga Island from the Kabaka in 1960. He justified his ownership of the island by defending British sleeping sickness control policy. He argued the previous island occupants had forfeited land rights by being diseased: "The island is a healthy place now. The British were correct to tell people to leave."[127] Another example of local people pursuing opportunities in sleeping sickness resettlement resulted from ambiguity about ultimate authority and tax collection in newly resettled areas. At Bugoto landing in Busoga, Ahamada Olwita placed sleeping sickness control as part of an ongoing process by the state of redirecting customary taxes away from local authority:

The fishing people used to ask my fathers for permission to build homes here, and gave my fathers gifts for using this beach—fish and other things. But then the beach was closed by the British, and when people came back, they said they had permission—that they were tested and given passes. The British Doctors did not ask me about these strangers. These people say they have to pay taxes to the government, so they don't ask my permission or give me what they should.[128]

Ahamada Olwita said the British closed the beach because of sickness, but that when they opened it again "they did not consider whose land it was before."

Ironically, the long-term result of sleeping sickness control in Uganda was a lack of African interest in resettlement. Many young people preferred to remain where they ended up after sleeping sickness removals. Continued restrictions on fishing, settlements reserved for men only, and requirements for physical examinations and passes alienated permanent resettlement. In 1922, 3,700 Bavuma resettled on the islands where 11,000 had been evicted 12 years prior. The total estimated population of Buvuma was down to 2,500 in 1947.[129] The estimated population of the Sesse Islands was 20,000 in 1900 and 5,000 in 1960.[130] In 1959 the Uganda Credit and Savings Bank denied settlers loans in southern Busoga because they considered land tenure there too insecure.[131] Without access to bank loans, farmers were less likely to settle and expand production. Land ownership was fluid, and settlers in the area were mobile. In 1963 only 33 percent of settlers in southern Busoga were Busogan, and 25 percent of farms had changed hands in the previous two years.[132] Africans were hesitant to invest in land with a history of unpredictable alienation, and instability and mobility continued. In Uganda, as in Tanzania, cycles of land alienation and resettlement resulted from the interaction between colonial sleeping sickness control policies and African responses to these policies.

DIAGNOSIS AND TREATMENT

> I was not yet married and very scared. This was the first white I had seen and he came close to me and called to me. He made me turn on my back to collect my blood. He did this from behind so I couldn't see what he was doing.
>
> Coletha Francisco[133]

Moments of disease policing—at fly pickets, during surveys and resettlement, and at labor camps—often involved medical examinations of blood tests, lymph smears, and spinal taps. Through the 1950s sleeping sickness treatment and diagnosis continued to have the same kind of bad reputation it had when connected to the "camps for the dead" in Uganda in the early part of the century. As with Coletha Francisco recalling a medical test, people feared and avoided diagnosis and drug treatment that since 1903 continued to be experimental, intrusive, and painful and have mixed results.

In 1953 a tsetse officer reported to the director of medical services that during his blood-slide survey of Kagunga village, "There were wild rumors of our blood thirsty intentions so people hide and evade over the borders and into the hills."[134] The officer sent a settlement scout out one day ahead of him to inform people to appear at the village in the early morning. He called names from existing census sheets and gave those in attendance metal disks with identification numbers to wear around their necks indicating they had been examined. He estimated up to 25 percent of residents were absent. Individuals then filed past medical assistants who felt for enlarged glands. Medical personnel took blood for blood slides from suspicious cases, and if glands were swollen enough to be punctured, they extracted gland juice. Of the 3,000 people the tsetse surveyor and his team examined in Kagunga during this eight-day visit, they took blood from 1,535. The team weighed those who they took blood from and then gave them prophylactic injections according to weight. The officer then held the residents for 30 minutes to "rest" and released them. The blood slides identified 46 new cases of sleeping sickness. The medical team gave these people lumbar punctures and drug injections and handed them over to the local native dresser for future treatments.[135]

Sleeping sickness officials complained that Africans often didn't report cases of sickness, that "their indifference to the disease is appalling."[136] But reporting a case elicited examinations and the surveillance by medical officials of everyone living near the victim.[137] And officers despaired that Africans avoided examinations, and that patients often abandoned treatment. Twenty-five of the 80 infected people whom sleeping sickness personnel identified in Runzewe between January 1944 and May 1945 disappeared after the initial examination.[138] Medical officials were then faced with the problem of losing track of potentially infectious patients.[139] Officials gave local chiefs the responsibility of controlling patients, or placed patients in hospitals for the duration of treatment. The threat of this kind of surveillance or incarceration caused further African resistance to medical examinations and treatment. A sleeping sickness scout in a Biharamulo village sent to transport three cases to the hospital reported in 1955 that he was physically attacked by one patient and that the local chief did nothing to help the scout with the patients.[140]

Drug treatments from the 1920s through the 1950s were long-term and had toxic side effects.[141] Colonial doctors never regularized drug treatment and continued to administer a complicated long-term series of injections. Complete treatment might bind Africans to a clinic for months. In 1933 the Tanganyika medical department recommended a month of treatment with Bayer 5 for cases diagnosed early. The department advocated injections on the 1st, 3rd, 5th, 8th, 15th, and 22nd days. For cases diagnosed late, treatment involved a 12-week series of injections of Bayer 5 combined with Tryparsamide extended to 20 weeks for relapsed cases.[142] In the 1950s doctors replaced Tryparsamide injections with Melarsen Oxide (known as Mel B).[143] All three of these drugs had toxic side affects. In 1955 the Nyakahura sleeping sickness camp assistant medical officer reported that antrypol injections had killed some healthy patients.[144]

Villagers did not know the purpose of visits by sleeping sickness officials beforehand. Even if they had previous experiences with sleeping sickness officers and scouts, there were numerous possible purposes of a visit. The sleeping sickness official might be there to announce relocation or new settlement rules, or to tell villagers they could expect new neighbors, or to make labor demands. He might be there for a simple inspection tour, or to perform medical examinations. Nor did sleeping sickness officials necessarily explain the purpose of the exams and treatment, and Tanzanians did not necessarily believe explanations if they were given.

Within settlements in both Tanganyika and Uganda, health workers were usually African employees of the health department not from local communities. Colonial departments trained and stationed African workers in settlements as fly guards, settlement guards, game department guards, teachers, and health clinic dressers. Native authorities were usually responsible for the maintenance of these workers, and the workers were dependent on local people for food, community, and carrying out their jobs.[145] Local people negotiated with and co-opted these employees. Outside African government employees quickly were drawn into local politics and power struggles, as they became part of settlement communities, and depended on local people for food and support. The Medical Department, for example, established a tribal dresser system in 1926 and trained, on average, 300 African dressers annually between 1930 and 1946. The department assigned dressers to clinics throughout the territory. A medical service memorandum from 1947 reported the dresser system was ineffective: "90% of dressers are useless from the medical point of view, having quite naturally degenerated from the effect of their surroundings into dishonest and incapable practitioners."[146] African dressers, for their part, complained of lack of medical supplies and adequate facilities, food, clothes, and direction from the state.[147]

African dressers in sleeping sickness settlements were poorly supplied colonial agents in remote communities. They negotiated their positions as strangers by forming relationships with local people, farmed to supplement their incomes, and used their relationship to the colonial state to become involved in local political issues.[148] Dressers are a further example of how the colonial idea of planned sleeping sickness settlements translated into African experiences unforeseen by colonial officers and beyond their control.

CONCLUSION

The creating and policing of sleeping sickness settlements and depopulated fly areas involved social, economic, and environmental interventions. In the 1930s British colonial officials began to locate sleeping sickness control in an inclusive system of development where economic, political, environmental, and physical health were all interdependent. They imagined settlements as places to modernize African behaviors. In the process of making boundaries between healthy and unhealthy space, sleeping sickness authorities attempted to control African movements and activities. In attempting to regulate the mobile, and therefore dangerous (in terms of human-fly contact), African economies of hunting, honey collecting, fishing, charcoal production, and iron smelting, sleeping sickness controls sought to survey and restructure African production within and between planned sleeping sickness settlements.

But while resettlement policies were meant to promote sustainable agriculture and longer-term African investment in land and community, African responses combined with minimum settlement population requirements to create further instability and insecurity regarding settlement patterns. In Uganda and Tanganyika, Africans successfully used a variety of strategies to resist colonial sleeping sickness resettlement and to adjust resettlement to their advantage. Colonial policy, in practice, was informed by Africans' politics, production systems, and preferences. Africans consistently rejected, or never considered, concentration as disease control. They did not separate colonial science and medicine from the broader historic context of colonial violence and power and focused instead on British expropriation of land and labor.

NOTES

1. Report on Karagwe Chiefdom, June 15, 1935, TNA, Dar es Salaam, 215/660; Preliminary Survey of Uzinza, May 1937, TNA 25102; Ikoma Sleeping Sickness Area Survey, July 1, 1942, TNA 463.

2. N. V. Rounce, *The Agriculture of the Cultivation Steepe of the Lake, Western, and Central Provinces* (Dar es Salaam, 1949), quoted in Ford, *African Ecology*, 230.

3. Tsetse Research Department Report, 1935–1938, TNA; Director Tsetse Research to District Commissioner Musoma, April 24, 1944, TNA 32535.

4. Sleeping Sickness Officer to Director of Medical Services, Dar es Salaam, September 1, 1945, TNA 28446; C. Macquarie to Sleeping Sickness Officer, Tabora, November 22, 1939, TNA 192/251; Anti-Sleeping Sickness Measures, Provincial Commissioner, Western Province, July 23, 1940, TNA 192/251.

5. H. M. O. Lester, "Sleeping Sickness Concentrations, Tanganyika Territory," 1938, Wellcome Medical Archive.

6. Moffett, "Strategic Retreat," 36–37.

7. Chief Aedalla to Sleeping Sickness Guard, June 3, 1944, TNA T5/2/107; Provincial Commissioner Western Province to District Commissioners, December 29, 1952, TNA P4/66, Vol. III.

8. Report on Plan Clearance and Settlement of Nyahunge-Isaka Valley, November 3, 1951, TNA 215 T5/3.

9. Sleeping Sickness Report Mwanza, June-August 1932, TNA 20909; G. Maclean, Sleeping Sickness Memorandum, September 8, 1927, TNA 19357.

10. Uganda Protectorate Annual Medical and Sanitary Report, 1936, ZA.

11. Acting Director of Tsetse Survey and Reclamation, February 2, 1953, TNA 29315; Tanganyika Tsetse Survey and Reclamation Department Annual Report, 1951, 15–16, TNA.

12. Fly Picket Returns, June 14–July 31, 1926, TNA 2702, Vol. II.

13. Fly Post Returns, Kasulu Post, 1954, TNA P4/62.

14. Tsetse Survey and Reclamation Department Annual Report, 1950, ZA; Acting Director of Tsetse Survey and Reclamation, February 2, 1953, TNA 29315.

15. Swynnerton to Chief Secretary, November 17, 1924, TNA 2702, Vol. II.; Swynnerton to Provincial Commissioner Tabora, January 20, 1927, TNA 2702, Vol. II. The substance was first developed to catch fleas on rats (plague).

16. Tsetse Control Meeting, November 20, 1933, TNA T5/1, Vol. I.

17. Mackenzie, *The Empire of Nature*, 242–243.

18. D. Anderson, "Depression, Dust Bowl, Demography, and Drought," 321–343.

19. McClintock, 208.

20. Fairbairn, 22.

21. Kjekshus, 178–179.

22. Sleeping Sickness Development Memo, June 1943, TNA 31731.

23. June 7, 1932 TNA 20763.

24. Settlement Officer Report, July 1957, Biharamulo, TNA T5 Vol. III.

25. Agriculture in Relation to Tsetse Reclamation, Wakefield, Director of Agriculture, March 23, 1933, TNA 21261, Vol. VII.

26. Maclean, "Sleeping Sickness Measures," 120–126.

27. Agricultural Officer Western Province to Provincial Commissioner, January 18, 1946, TNA 28936.

28. Provincial Commissioner Lake to Director of Medicine and Sanitation, January 30, 1935, TNA 1022 Vol. I.

29. Draft Memorandum on the Establishment of Controlled Settlement Areas, Provincial Commissioner Western Province, May 4, 1951, TNA 192/251.

30. Agriculture in Relation to Tsetse Reclamation, Wakefield, Director of Agriculture, March 23, 1933, TNA 21261, Vol. VII.; Maclean, "Sleeping Sickness Measures," 123–124.

31. Provincial Commissioner Western Province to Chief Secretary, January 3, 1934, TNA 21711.

32. Lester, 8.

33. Provincial Commissioner Western Province to Chief Secretary, February 12, 1934, TNA 21711.

34. Provincial Commissioner Western Province to CMS, May 2, 1934, TNA 21711.

35. Director of Education to Chief Secretary, July 11, 1934, TNA 21711.

36. H. Langford, CMS Uha to Bishop Central Tanganyika, June 18, 1934, TNA 21711; also see Beck, *A History of British Medical Administration*, 120–122.

37. Lester, 7.

38. Population Map, 1936, TNA 192/215.

39. Draft Memorandum on the Establishment of Controlled Settlement Areas, Provincial Commissioner Western Province, May 4, 1951, TNA 192/251.

40. C. Macquirie, Runzewe Survey, May 29, 1945, TNA, Dar es Salaam, 192/215.

41. Sleeping Sickness Survey Northwest Tabora, November 11, 1950, TNA P4/66 Vol. III.

42. Nguruka Survey, July 1953, TNA P4/66 Vol. II.

43. Tanganyika Territorial Tsetse Committee Meeting Minutes, October 16, 1947, TNA 28936.

44. Uganda Sleeping Sickness Ordinance, 1928, UNA; Sukuma Development Officer Report Geita, October 23, 1953, TNA T5/3 Vol. III.

45. C. Macquirie to Sleeping Sickness Officer Tabora, May 29, 1945, TNA 192/215; Agricultural Officer to Provincial Commissioner Western, January 18, 1946, TNA 192/215.

46. Memorandum on the Establishment of Controlled Settlement Areas, Provincial Commissioner Western Province, May 4, 1951, TNA 192/215.

47. Kibondo Settlement Report, January-August 1957, TNA P4/64 Vol. II.

48. Memorandum on the Establishment of Controlled Settlement Areas, Provincial Commissioner Western Province, May 4, 1951, TNA 192/215.

49. Nguruka Survey, July 1953, TNA P4/66 Vol. II.

50. Provincial Commissioner Lake to District Officers, July 30, 1949, TNA 192/215.

51. Provincial Office Meeting Tabora, November 28, 1950, TNA P4/61; Sleeping Sickness Report, Western Province, November 1954, TNA P4/64, Vol. II.

52. Sigulu Island Sleeping Sickness Rules, April 16, 1956, UNA.

53. Uganda Department of Health and Sanitation Annual Report, 1923, UNA.

54. Soff, "A History of Sleeping Sickness," 191–192.

55. Uganda Department of Health and Sanitation Annual Report, 1920, 64, UNA; Sagitu Island Sleeping Sickness Rules, 1956, UNA.

56. Uganda Department of Health and Sanitation Annual Report, 1937, 34, UNA.

57. Uha and Kahama Development Report, 1933, TNA 21712, Vol. III

58. District Officer Bukoba to Provincial Commissioner Mwanza, December 29, 1935, TNA 215/660, Vol. III.

59. Provincial Commissioner Lake Province to Chief Secretary, June 8, 1943, TNA 28446.

60. Interview with Mukama Nakuringa, Biharamulo, Tanzania, October 12, 1994.

61. Interview with Salvatory Kalema, Katoro, Tanganyika, September 16, 1994.

62. Group Interview, Biharamulo, Tanganyika, November 10, 1994.

63. J. E. S. Lamb to Provincial Commissioner Lake Province, January 21, 1955, TNA T5/126/6.

64. Men and Women of Nyakamwaga to District Commissioner, Mwanza, November 9, 1934, TNA T5/126/7.

65. Interview with Bazage Kanumi, Biharamulo, Tanzania, September 30, 1994.

66. Mwami Kandege to District Commissioner Mpanda, March 3, 1957, TNA 192/251.

67. Quarterly Meeting of Chiefs, April 1942, TNA 192/251.

68. Mrisho Migila to District Commissioner Tabora, May 16, 1955, TNA P4/66, Vol. IV.

69. District Commissioner Mpanda to Baraza Ukonongo, October 15, 1951, TNA P4/66, Vol. II.

70. Provincial Commissioner Southern to Director of Medical Services, May 28, 1938, TNA 12698; Kapele Ngugulu to Sleeping Sickness Officer Tabora, July 11, 1952, TNA P4/66, Vol. III.; District Officer Musoma to Provincial Commissioner Lake Province, Nov. 29, 1950, TNA 463; Sleeping Sickness Officer to Director Tsetse Research Shinyanga, May 7, 1935, TNA 1022, Vol. III.

71. Report on Bwanga-Busonzo Concentrations, Agricultural Surveyor, July 30, 1939, TNA 192/251.

72. Concentration at Ushirombo, Assistant District Officer Kahama, May 13, 1942, TNA 192/251.

73. Selemani Ikamazya to District Commissioner Tabora, June 10, 1953, TNA P466, Vol. III.

74. Report for Geita, 1939, Agricultural Surveyor, TNA 1022, Vol. I.

75. Meeting Technical Officers Medical, Veterinary, Tsetse and Agricultural Departments, Mwanza, November 20, 1933, TNA T5/1 Vol. II.

76. District Commissioner Mpunze to Provincial Commissioner Western, October 26, 1940, TNA 192/251.

77. C. Macquarie to Sleeping Sickness Officer Tabora, November 22, 1939, TNA 192/251.

78. Report on Bwanga-Busonzo Concentrations, Agricultural Surveyor, July 30, 1939, TNA 192/251.

79. District Commissioner Nzega to Provincial Commissioner Tabora, April 6, 1951, TNA 192/251.

80. Interview with Rutekelayo Ifunza, Katoro Village, Geita, Tanzania, September 16, 1994.

81. People of Buyombe to District Officer Mwanza, November 9, 1934, TNA 215/660.

82. C. Macquarie to Sleeping Sickness Officer Tabora, November 22, 1939, TNA 192/251.

83. Selemani Ikamazya to District Commissioner Tabora, June 10, 1953, TNA 466, Vol. III.

84. Minutes of the Quarterly Meeting of Chiefs, April 1942, TNA 192/251.

85. District Commissioner to Provincial Commissioner Lake Province, September 27, 1951, TNA 215 T5/3 Vol. III

86. Deputy District Commissioner Geita to District Commissioner Geita, October 19, 1951, TNA 215 T5/3 Vol. III.

87. Ibid.

88. Provincial Commissioner to District Commissioner, September 27, 1951, TNA, 215/T5/3 Vol. III.

89. Edward, Vincent, Orwochi, Jolam to Provincial Commissioner Mwanza, September 15, 1951, TNA 215 T5/3 Vol. III.

90. District Commissioner to Patel and Patel, Mwanza, September 12, 1951, TNA.

91. Provincial Commissioner to Edward, Vincent, Orwochi, Jolam, November 6, 1951, TNA.

92. District Commissioner Geita to Provincial Commissioner Lake, August 1, 1951, TNA 215 T5/3, Vol. III.

93. Provincial Commissioner Lake Minutes, June 29, 1953, TNA 215 T5/3 Vol. III; District Commissioner to Vincent Olutoch, November 1,1953, TNA 215 T5/3 Vol. III.

94. Vincent Olutoch to Chief Native Commissioner, Dar es Salaam, May 20, 1953, TNA 215 T5/3 Vol. III.

95. District Commissioner to Provincial Commissioner Lake, March 14, 1956, TNA 215 T5/3 Vol. III.

96. Provincial Commissioner Lake to Local Government Office, April 6, 1956, TNA 215 T5/3 Vol. III.

97. Interview with Brighton Ogongo, Buyanga, Sigulu Island, December 10, 1993.

98. Busoga Resettlement Report, March 1926, Secretariat Minute 7013, and Busoga Sleeping Sickness Area Tour Report, January 1909, Secretariat Minute 2047, UNA, Entebbe.

99. Mahmood Mamdani, *Politics and Class Formation in Uganda* (New York, 1976), 171.

100. Letter from Citizens of Bomba Island to District Officer, February 1926, Secretariat Minute 7013, UNA.

101. Land Dispute Report, September 1926, Secretariat Minute 7013, UNA.

102. Ibid.

103. Uganda Protectorate Annual Medical and Sanitary Report, (1920), ZA.

104. Southern Busoga Sub-District Report for 1952, Wellcome Medical Library, London.

105. Bruce, 56.

106. Mackichan, 49–51.

107. Worthington, *Development Plan.*

108. Barnley, 264–265; Watts, 10.

109. J. T. Fleming, Kiterera Resettlement Report, July-August 1956, BDA.

110. South Busoga Resettlement Report, February 1960, BDA.

111. J. T. Fleming, Kiterera Resettlement Report, January 1956, BDA.

112. Ibid.

113. Watts, 19–20.

114. Mamdani, 196.

115. J. T. Fleming, April 1956, BDA.

116. J. T. Fleming, June 1957, BDA.

117. J. T. Fleming, March 1956 and February 1957, BDA.

118. Group Interview, Biharamulo, Tanganyika, November 10, 1994.

119. J. T. Fleming, February 1957, BDA.

120. J. T. Fleming, June 1957, BDA.

121. D. H. H. Robertson, "Trypanosomiasis in South-East Uganda," 628.

122. Uganda Tsetse Control Department Annual Report, 1950, ZA.

123. Soff, "A History of Sleeping Sickness," 215–216.

124. D. H. H. Robertson, "Trypanosomiasis in South-East Uganda," 635.

125. Personal Correspondences, Brighton O. and District Commissioner, May-July 1963, BDA.

126. Brighton Correspondence, July 27, 1963, BDA.

127. Interview with Alexander Salongo Mugenyi, Mpuga Island, Uganda, January 25, 1995.

128. Interview with Ahamada Olwita Bugoto, Iganga, Uganda, November 10–13, 1993.

129. Southern Busoga Sub-District Report, 1953, Wellcome Medical Library, London.

130. A. M. O'Connor, *An Economic Geography of East Africa* (London, 1966); Annual Medical and Sanitary Report for the Year Ended 31st December 1922 (Entebbe, 1923).

131. Watts, 21.

132. Ibid., 26.

133. Interview with Coletha Francisco, Katoro Village, Geita, Tanzania, September 17, 1994.

134. Tsetse Officer Kibondo to Director Medical Services, December 18, 1953, TNA, P4/64/II.

135. Tsetse Officer Kibondo to Director Medical Services, December 18, 1953, TNA, P4/64/II.

136. Provincial Commissioner to District Commissioners Lake Province, July 30, 1949, TNA 192/215.

137. Report on Sleeping Sickness in Buganda, Buchosa, Provincial Tsetse Officer Mwanza, April 30, 1949, TNA T5/3 215.

138. C. Macquirie to Sleeping Sickness Officer Tabora, May 29, 1945, TNA 192/215.

139. Assistant Medical Officer, Nyakahura Sleeping Sickness Camp, to Director Medical Services, July 15, 1954, TNA, 251/192.

140. Sleeping Sickness Guard to District Officer, November 12, 1955, TNA T5/II.

141. Treatment Report, Sleeping Sickness Officer, Tabora, TNA T5/2; Assistant Medical Officer, Nayakahura Sleeping Sickness Camp to Director Medical Services, July 15, 1954, TNA 251/192.

142. G. Maclean, *Sleeping Sickness Notes* (Dar es Salaam: Tanganyika Territory Medical Department, 1933), 2–7.

143. Treatment Report, Sleeping Sickness Officer, Tabora, TNA, T5/2.

144. Assistant Medical Officer, Nyakahura Sleeping Sickness Camp, to Director Medical Services, July 15, 1954, TNA, 251/192.

145. Neumann, *Imposing Wilderness.*

146. Memorandum on Rural Medical Services, Director of Medical Services, December 6, 1947, TNA 21710.

147. Ibid.

148. Geita Dresser Reports, May-August 1948, TNA 21710.

CHAPTER 6

Labor, Land, and Colonial Disease Control

I am informed that the turn out of labor, if not voluntary as we know the meaning of the word, is at least recognized by natives as part of the ordinary routine of their year.

Sleeping Sickness Officer F. Longland[1]

Every person always has a choice. But in deciding to go to work or not, people thought about the consequences of going against the head of the family, chief or white person.

Bazage Kanumi[2]

Bush clearing and resettlement were the two primary methods of tsetse control in the British East African colonies. British colonial scientists organized these two methods to work in tandem. Cleared tsetse barriers protected resettled villages, and concentrated populations added to barrier fronts by maintaining cleared agricultural lands. African labor, primarily unpaid, constructed tsetse barriers of various sizes and shapes throughout Tanganyika and Uganda in the colonial period. Different kinds of clearings had different environmental and socioeconomic effects and reflected particular British ideological relationships to African lands and people.

Colonialists and Africans both recognized the moral and legal tensions between policies of forced labor for brush clearing, forced depopulations and land expropriation, and the rhetorics associated with the civilizing mission, development, and disease control. Sleeping sickness control policies contradicted central premises of Western capitalism and modernity such as private property and free labor. Western debates about forced labor continued throughout the colonial period. State directives to district officials about raising labor in Kenya in 1919 generated political scandal in Britain and Kenya. Frederick Cooper argues that the British government considered itself progressive on the issue of colonial labor. The British were on the forefront of promoting the international Forced Labour Convention in 1930. The primary focus of this agreement was to regulate the recruitment and treatment of African labor by private enterprise and to differentiate between free and forced labor. In the resulting agreement forced labor was legitimate as an "exceptional measure." What constituted an exceptional measure remained vague, but for the British it came to include public works, disease control, and agricultural development work.[3] Officials' writings about Africans' relationships to land and work reflected debates about the legality and morality of forced labor. Such debates framed how they represented forced labor to themselves and to Africans. There was a great distance between local African and colonial understandings of the rationale behind brush-clearing labor. Local people's understandings were produced through their experiences with colonial power in general and brush clearing in particular. Also African responses to sleeping sickness control took on meanings within the context of colonial debates about coercion and land alienation, and some local people benefited from tensions in colonial ideology and practice.

Colonialists were concerned about justifying coercion as a civilized and moral practice to themselves and to colonized people. Throughout the colonial debates on forced labor, arguments that it was justified were based on the particularities of African backwardness.[4] Paternalist conversations justifying coercion as part of sleeping sickness control argued that control policies were for Africans' own good and that Africans were partially to blame for the spread of tsetse and for a myriad of environmental problems. The other side of the arguments justifying force was that the coercion wasn't oppressive, that Africans did not really mind forced resettlement and brush clearing, and that Africans usually agreed to resettle and to volunteer their labor according to British directions.

Restrictions on the movement of Africans in sleeping sickness areas and use of male labor for brush clearing was also at odds with a constant British demand for African labor on public works, plantations, and in urban areas in Uganda and Tanganyika. Sleeping sickness controls impacted the movement of labor within and across colonial boundaries and the surveillance of labor on mines and plantations near tsetse areas.

In a rhetoric that extends to the present, colonialists addressed the issue of long-term land alienation, and the seeming failure of control policies to impede the spread of tsetse, by arguing that the value of Africa was in its flora and fauna and that Africans destroyed African nature. The colonial story of sleeping sickness control told that the colonial state would hold depopulated fly lands temporarily in trust until local people were capable of winning them back from tsetse. By the 1930s an alternative narrative emerged that used the overarching value of nature conservation to champion tsetse as the protectors of African environments. According to this logic, Africans were aggressors against environmental order, and sleeping sickness and the state alienation of land were the just and necessary price they paid for transience, lack of erosion control, and the lack of political and economic order. Tsetse were saving nature from African mismanagement, and the state permanently alienated some fly areas by declaring them nature reserves. As this history of colonial sleeping sickness control began with the overlapping geographies of Ganda-British imperialism and tsetse areas in Uganda, the long-term implications of sleeping sickness controls in Uganda and Tanganyika are reflected in the overlapping geographies of former tsetse-control areas and current national parks.

BRUSH CLEARING IN TANGANYIKA

Discussions about coercion, free choice, and African culpability in the presence of disease influenced the practice of forced brush clearing. The Tsetse Department published a series of general guidelines for the organization of clearing labor from the 1930s through the 1950s. In practice, tsetse officers deployed labor in a variety of ways depending on local conditions and available resources and adjusting to African actions and demands. But clearing actions did follow a general pattern. Initially, tsetse officers directed chiefs to instruct adult men to assemble at a certain place and time and to bring their own tools and food for the required number of workdays. If the barrier was nearby, laborers could commute daily. More often, however, the extent of required labor meant tsetse officers marched or transported by truck tribal turnouts to labor camps where workers lived while clearing vegetation. Tsetse officers usually requested chiefs to assemble one-third to one-half of all adult men.[5]

Specially trained tsetse labor prepared clearing sites by placing sighting poles, using army compasses, and clearing two-foot-wide border lines.[6] When voluntary labor arrived on site, Tsetse Department guidelines from 1932 recommended that officers organize them into work gangs of 25 men under the supervision of headmen wearing caps and armbands for easy identification. Gangs were to work closely together, one man per yard, as "they work more happily when close together."[7] White officers supervised a maximum of 500 workers each. The Tsetse Department supplied work camps with buckets for drinking water, a truck and fuel for transportation, and a rifle and ammunition for protection from animals and to provide meat. All available blacksmiths settled into camps with their equipment to repair broken tools, and native dressers from the nearest clinics relocated to staff medical stations.[8]

In the 1930s discriminative brush clearing became the primary focus of research at Shinyanga and the practiced method of choice throughout British Africa. The detailed mapping and surveillance involved in controlling settlements and African mobility was also required for precise discriminative brush clearing. British scientists emphasized that discriminative clearing was the most sophisticated and advanced means of tsetse control. Discriminative clearing required the greatest degree of entomological and botanical knowledge and the most precise use of African labor. As an example, the project to eliminate tsetse from 300 square miles between Arusha and Moshi in 1943 involved clearing 26 small, defined vegetation communities (see figure 6.1).[9] The clearing scheme for the Singida Hexagon plan begun in 1936 called for an 8-mile defense in depth around the 19-mile hexagon perimeter. This included a total of 152 square miles, of which, according to the methods of discriminatory clearing, 25 square miles would have to be actually

Figure 6.1
Map of Discriminative Clearings near Arusha, Tanganyika, 1943

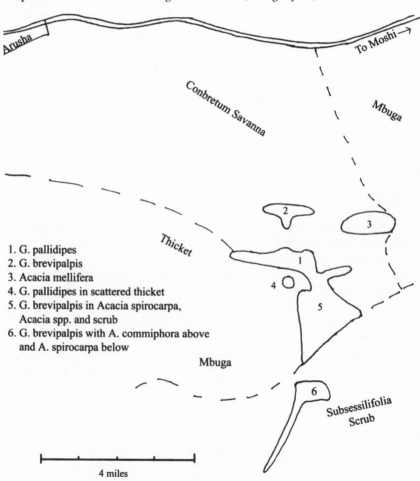

1. G. pallidipes
2. G. brevipalpis
3. Acacia mellifera
4. G. pallidipes in scattered thicket
5. G. brevipalpis in Acacia spirocarpa,
   Acacia spp. and scrub
6. G. brevipalpis with A. commiphora above
   and A. spirocarpa below

4 miles

Based on a map in TNA 215/T5/3, 1943.

cleared.[10] Discriminative clearing also addressed British ideological hesitations about sheer clearing, a method which created the kind of visual desolation the British were trying to overcome. An East African Tsetse and Trypanosomiasis Research and Reclamation Organization Report from 1949 argued sheer clearing was a mistake, as "the general aspect is one of ghastly desolation."[11] The dominant late-nineteenth- and early-twentieth-century English idea about parkland was that natural scenery should be preserved, restored, and enhanced, as opposed to completely restructured.[12] Discriminative clearing was an expression of esthetic and conservationist ideas in tsetse control, as it left nature partially intact and accessible.

According to colonial statistics for Tanganyika, by 1944 African men had worked 2.25 million man-days to clear approximately 500 square miles, resulting in the reclamation of a total of 1,000 square miles.[13] By 1960 tsetse barriers had reclaimed an additional 1,000 square miles. Until World War II, most of the clearing was sheer, and after 1945, most was discriminative.[14] Close to 80 percent of the total tsetse territory reclaimed by clearing was in the Lake Victoria basin—in the Lake, Central, and Western Provinces.[15]

Colonial clearing schemes called for much more clearing than was ever accomplished and more labor than could be raised. The Singida Hexagon plan begun in 1936 called for an 8-mile defense in depth around the 19-mile hexagon perimeter and 250,000 man-days of labor. As tsetse bush in Tanganyika continued to expand in spite of clearing efforts, so did the scale of proposed clearing schemes and labor demands. Musoma schemes in 1944 called for 200,000 man-days in the form of 4,000 men for 10 days of labor per year for five years.[16] There were six major clearing schemes in Lake Province alone in 1946. In 1947 the Tanganyikan colonial labor commission complained that sleeping sickness labor requested by clearing scheme plans in Central Province alone was 10 percent of the total territorial labor force working on sisal plantations and 50 percent of the total labor force employed in mining.[17]

TSETSE BARRIERS IN UGANDA

The colonial government in Uganda established a Tsetse Control Department in 1947. The focus on tsetse control was in northern and central Uganda and along Lake Victoria, again away from the core of the Gandan state. Tsetse-control officers replaced early methods of sleeping sickness depopulations to stop epidemics, with tsetse control as a preventative action necessary to assure future development. Governor John Hall wrote in the introduction to the 1946 Uganda Development Plan that without massive fly control efforts, "there can be no economic or social future for Uganda."[18]

Tsetse surveys in Uganda in the 1940s identified expanding fly fronts and large regions of tsetse infestation. As in Tanganyika, reclamation schemes involved fly barriers of various sizes, shapes, and types to block fly advances into development areas (see figure 6.2). But while discriminative clearing and controlled burning was a component of barrier clearing in Uganda, environmental and political differences from Tanganyika placed tsetse control in Uganda on a separate course.

Game destruction was a primary method of tsetse reclamation in colonial Uganda. The Tsetse Control Department employed white and African hunters to shoot specific species of game in designated tsetse barriers. Tsetse officials targeted buffalo, bushbuck, and bushpigs, but tsetse-control hunters also killed rhinos, elephants, and crocodiles.[19] By 1954 the Tsetse Control Department employed and equipped 250 African hunters.[20] Hunters swept barrier areas and were stationed along barrier boundaries to prevent game movements. In North Mengo between 1945 and 1952, hunters reported shooting 15,000 animals.[21] In western Bunyoro between 1951 and 1956, hunters reported shooting 13,000 animals.[22]

In tsetse barriers, hunting was usually combined with discriminative clearing, controlled burning, and densification. Tsetse officials reported burning and clearing efforts alone often failed. Environmental conditions made clearing vegetation particularly difficult in much of Uganda. By the 1940s, tsetse were spreading primarily through areas of tall grass and seasonal swamps.[23] Tsetse areas in Uganda were relatively wetter than in Tanganyika. Tsetse officers in Ankole in 1950 reported that controlled burning had failed because there was too much rain.[24] Ugandan tsetse areas were also more densely forested, so more difficult to access and clear even with discriminative methods. Some tsetse researchers in Uganda argued, in fact, that tall, dense grass, untrampled and unburned (densification), was a valuable fly barrier. In 1949 in northern Uganda, tsetse hunters targeted rhinos and elephant herds, as scientists believed large game created fly access corridors by trampling tall grass. Hunters shot 18 elephants in the area in 1950 and all 12 black rhinos.[25]

Labor relations in Uganda were also different from Tanganyika. The Tsetse Department did not rely on unpaid tribal turnouts, but used paid labor and prison labor for clearing. There was a precolonial history in Uganda of farmers owing landlords and chiefs some material tribute and labor.[26] With the Uganda Agreement in 1900, the British initiated a system of labor known as *kasanvu* obliging Ugandans to do 30 days compulsory labor for the government if they could not pay taxes in cash. The colonial state used the *kasanvu* system to raise large labor parties to build the Kampala sewage system and railway lines. Ugandans resisted *kasanvu* labor through out-migration, and the system depressed wages in a period when the colonial state was trying to attract wage labor and promote cash-crop production. The British abandoned the state forced-labor system in Uganda in 1927 and the labor tribute requirements to local chiefs in 1936.[27] By the 1940s there was no existing precedent for colonial demands of unpaid labor. Unlike in Tanganyika, where there was ideological and political space to create a tradition of forced labor, in Uganda the colonial state had already used and then moved away from this

Figure 6.2
Map of Tsetse Advances and Barriers, Uganda, 1960

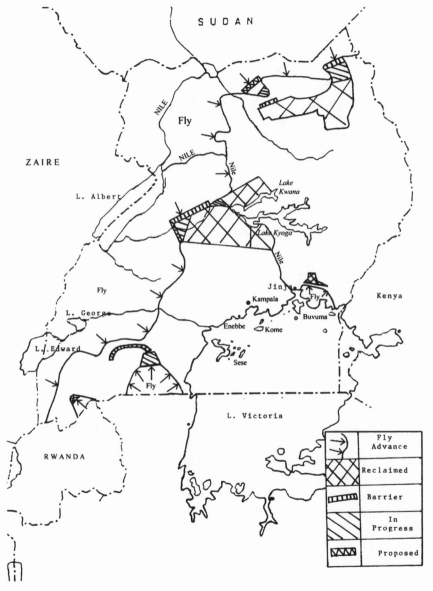

Uganda Tsetse Control Department Annual Report, 1960, UNA.

practice. After 1936 Ugandan workers expected to be paid for government work.

The Tsetse Control Department organized labor into smaller mechanized units. Clearing teams were organized with vehicles, cooks, hunters (to provide meat), and "ax-men" moving methodically through proscribed areas.[28] In the 1950s the Tsetse Department in Uganda was at the forefront of insecticide use. "Spray units" used truck-, boat-, and knapsack-mounted sprayers to apply dieldrin and DDT solutions to vegetation cover along "spray barriers."[29]

The colonial state's relationship to labor was also connected to its relationship to game control and conservation. The Uganda colonial state early on conflicted with conservation advocates. Before World War I, colonial officials in Uganda complained that game reserves were too large and that game—particularly buffalo, elephants, and pigs later targeted in tsetse control—were destroying farms and threatening agricultural production in large areas of Ankole and Toro in northern Uganda.[30] The state supported game destruction in defense of agricultural productivity against pressure from British conservationists. The state was committed to protecting local farmers from nature, not to protecting nature from farmers. By the 1940s the colonial state was even more firmly allied with, and dependent on, independent, small-scale cash-crop production in Uganda. Tsetse control as game destruction not only minimized disruptions of local farming, but actively promoted farming through the destruction of marauding game.

Conservationists bitterly denounced tsetse-control-mandated game destruction in Uganda. A. G. Robertson, a tsetse researcher in Uganda, acknowledged this criticism and bemoaned the fact: "This is a distasteful method of control, and no one would be happier than the government and the tsetse control department if it could be feasibly dispensed with." He offered that certain species—leopard, impala, and zebra—would not be hunted. But, he argued, all alternatives to game destruction had been tried. Previous attempts at bush clearing had failed "despite valiant efforts." Game control was cheap and effective in relation to the resources the colonial government had at hand and was necessary in face of "the extreme urgency of the situation—which certainly allows no time for the creation of any sort of barrier to further tsetse advance by bush clearing."[31]

The Tsetse Control Department continued to give primary responsibility for reclamation successes to game destruction and continued to rely on hunting to maintain tsetse barriers. Tsetse Department statistics credited game destruction with 5,000 of the 7,000 square miles reclaimed from tsetse in Uganda between 1947 and 1963.[32] Tsetse barriers in Uganda looked different from those in Tanganyika, and the Tsetse Control Department constructed them in different ways. Tsetse-control officers in Uganda used much less labor and boasted to have reclaimed much more land. African hunters shot game in tsetse barriers, but Ugandan labor did little clearing of vegetation.

FORCED LABOR

Colonial officials reported that they gave local people a choice in resettlement and that brush-clearing labor was voluntary; that way colonialism avoided coercion. Sleeping sickness officials would call village meetings, or *barazas*, where they would explain the policy of resettlement to local people. At *barazas*, they would explain how resettlement was for the good of the community and colony and invite everyone to agree to resettle. In colonialist texts, sleeping sickness *barazas* were signifiers of democratic process and African free choice. But colonial practice did not offer local people a choice between relocating and not relocating. For colonial officials at *barazas*, relocation was a given. Colonialists considered African rejections of the sleeping sickness story, and refusals to move or refusals to move to the location chosen by a colonial official, as evidence of African primitiveness and unscientific thinking that then necessitated and justified force.

Brush-clearing male labor was an integral component of tsetse control in Tanganyika from the beginning of 1923. Colonial analysis of African responses to tsetse-control labor and settlement demands were part of the core research questions at Shinyanga, and Swynnerton considered results of labor experiments vital to the feasibility of control methods. He wrote from Shinyanga, "It was decided to attempt at the outset to ascertain (i) whether an annual voluntary out turn of a native population could be organized to attack their own problems; (ii) whether natives could be persuaded to settle in places in which their presence would consolidate gains made or assist in making them." All experiments involved regrouping people, reforming African behaviors, and organizing voluntary labor "to attack their own problems."[33] British tsetse officers needed voluntary African labor to clear and burn bush, fight fires, and agree to live in certain areas and not in others.

The process of raising and controlling labor was a primary point of contention and negotiation between tsetse-control officers and local Africans. From the beginning of fly clearings in the early 1920s, the tsetse officers grappled with the issue of forced versus voluntary labor. It was important in British colonial Africa (and in Britain ideologically, economically, and politically in terms of the British ideas of informal rule and of sleeping sickness control as altruistic) that tsetse labor be perceived of as voluntary, as both for and by Africans: "The great thing is that the native is learning to tackle his own problem, and he knows that he is doing so himself and gains confidence from that fact."[34] Economically, the various departments involved did not have the money to pay clearing labor. Politically, the colonial state was concerned about the African resistance forced labor might generate. F. A. Montague, the tsetse reclamation officer of Northern Province, wrote in 1926, "In work of this sort any suspicion of unpaid labor should be scrupulously avoided."[35] It was important to the European presentation and successful implementation of colonial sleeping sickness control that Africans took on policy goals as their own.

To gather voluntary labor effectively, tsetse officers relied on unpaid, local labor turnouts (referred to by the British as "tribal-turnouts") organized by local leaders. Under a system of indirect rule, beginning in the 1920s tsetse officers gave local African leaders the responsibility for gathering groups of men for bush clearing work. Drawing on the logic of indirect rule, colonial officials pointed out that East African elite had traditional rights to make regular demands of unpaid communal labor for community projects and to maintain leaders' homes, fields, and livestock. Frederick Cooper argues that British indirect rule "serenely distanced officials from the messy world in which power was brought to bear on young men."[36] Although the tribal-turnout wasn't voluntary labor in a literal sense, tsetse officials justified using this labor by recasting the definition of force within their understanding of an African context as "at least recognized by natives as part of the ordinary routine of their year."

In Tanganyika, publications by the Tsetse Research Department show disease-control officers redefining the idea of force and maneuvering for African cooperation. They presented sleeping sickness control as a war of survival and national pride. Survey reports and fly maps used military vocabulary and imagery. An article in the *Uganda Journal* in 1935 was titled, "Mankind at War with the Insects," with subheadings, "The Enemy," "The Attack," "The Casualties," "Our Allies," "The Intelligence," and "Our Weapons."[37] This was an invasion with fly fronts, frontlines, advances and retreats by people and tsetse, flanking actions, and overrun positions (see figure 6.3).[38] Colonial texts compared the director of tsetse research and reclamation to an army commander with "his executive troops (reclamation side) and his intelligence department (scientific side)."[39] Charles Swynnerton wrote that the people of Shinyanga, "till we turned them, were definitely 'on the run.'" Swynnerton reported that he told alarmed Sukuma in Shinyanga to "stand firm and yourselves attack."[40] He praised the Shinyanga chief Makwaia for making "fighting speeches to his people in which the tsetse was described as the enemy, and themselves as soldiers in action."[41] The presentation of sleeping sickness control as a war of African armies and European advisers against tsetse served a variety of purposes. It justified colonial rule as in behalf of African interests to help Africans protect and eventually take back their own lands. It presented the war as ultimately a protonationalist conflict between Africans and invading flies, with British scientists as allies. It cast Africans' responses in the parameters of loyalty and treason, not to the colonial state, but to their own communities and ways of life: "Any slackening of effort is madness, and it should be everyone's duty, under such circumstances, to participate in the work."[42] According to the war analogy, people in fly areas had a patriotic duty to fight tsetse.

Swynnerton praised the cooperation of African labor in his early clearing operation in Shinyanga, but his descriptions of labor turnouts emphasized that the key to successfully organized African labor lay with local power re-

Figure 6.3
Map of Tsetse Advances and Barriers around Singida, Tanganyika, 1949

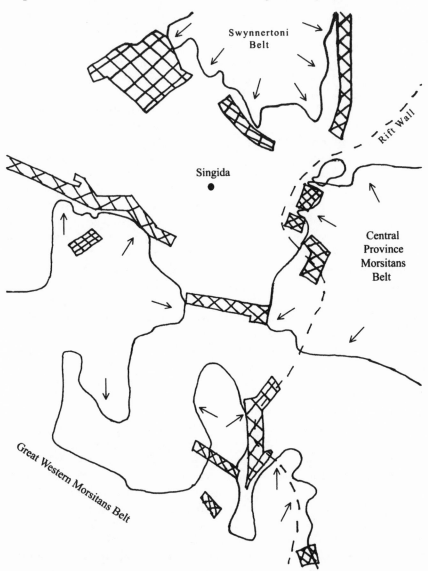

Based on a map in TNA 215/T5/3, 1949.

lations and respect for native authority. He named particularly dedicated and inspiring Shinyanga chiefs who were able to raise large labor parties, "especially, poor, blind Masanja, of Mondo, who, despite his infirmity, never left his workers."[43] It was less important for Swynnerton that Africans understood the scientific ideas behind sleeping sickness control plans than that British-organized bush clearing worked with and reinforced an effective, indigenous African social order: "Propaganda on these subjects is, relatively speaking, useless in respect of the adult native."[44] On the other hand, "prospects of effective co-operation have been lessened where it has been the policy to weaken or ignore their tribal organization."[45] Swynnerton's analysis of sleeping sickness conditions and controls revealed Africans were not only victims of disease, but were victims of political mismanagement, both by African elite and Europeans.

In this way, Swynnerton presented sleeping sickness control as a mechanism for establishing correct political order. As he saw it, part of the disease problem in Tanganyika was simply a lack of effective central authority and control. Swynnerton blamed colonial authority, in part, for not enforcing a political order necessary for effective environmental control. In his 1925 article, "The Tsetse-Fly Problem in the Nzega Sub-District," he linked tsetse-control schemes to the ideology of British indirect rule. Swynnerton connected local histories of tsetse-control successes and failures to just or oppressive chiefs. As an example for British rule he argued, "The chief lesson for ourselves in this region consists in the fact that an unpopular chieftain may cause the depopulation of an area and a consequent up-growth of bush and influx of tsetse."[46] He gave examples of Sultan Siyota who "oppressed his own people," thus causing "the depopulation of a piece of cultivation steppe." The British therefore justly deposed and deported him. Swynnerton goes on to give another example of a sultan who "engaged the people near him in such extensive works that they regarded them as hardship, and his immediate neighborhood also became deserted and grew up into tsetse infested bush."[47] By identifying oppressive chiefs, and pointing out villagers' willingness to tolerate them, Swynnerton blamed African behavior for the spread of tsetse and emphasized the need for the British to intervene in African politics when necessary.

Effective tsetse control, in contrast, and cooperation with British efforts were reflections of legitimate rule by wise elite: "We had conferences with the Sultans, and I was most struck with these hereditary native rulers of the district, with their information and outlook, their apparent ability and hold over their people, their ready grasp of the matter in hand and their shrewd suggestions, and their keenness to support the Government in an effective tackling of the outbreak."[48] Swynnerton presented sleeping sickness policies as legitimate because local African authorities supported them, and he presented local authorities as legitimate because they supported disease control plans.

By giving local leaders responsibility for raising labor and relocating people, colonial sleeping sickness control created and reified East African systems of traditional political authority. Furthermore, according to the logic of indirect rule, local people disobeying "native authority" were acting against natural African political order and being disloyal. So even if the argument of disease control as in Africans' best interests did not completely assuage the concerns of colonial officers and European popular opinion about coercion, colonial authors argued that critics could not legitimately hold force in Africa to the same moral scrutiny they held it in the West.

BLAMING AFRICANS

Colonialists mitigated the contradiction of colonial coercion by emphasizing Africans as agents, as well as victims, of disease. By categorizing African behaviors that exposed them to sleeping sickness and tsetse as backward, British scientists emphasized that primitive people were responsible for disease. Scientific texts argued Africans were unable to consolidate cultivation fronts, and that backward behaviors, such as mobility and disorganized brush burning, promoted the spread of tsetse. Sleeping sickness was evidence of primitiveness as unhealthy: "By the very nature of the disease the people at risk are the most backward natives in the Territory, those who live at the bare subsistence level, who are not interested in or affected by higher economic standards."[49] The battle against sleeping sickness became synonymous with battles against primitive land use and transience. Sleeping sickness scientists' discussions about sleeping sickness control presented "bush villages" as primitive because they were potentially tsetse infested. Africans, by choosing to live in the bush, abdicated certain human rights and legal claims.

This justified a spectrum of controls on behavior, production, and settlement patterns: "Once the bush village is compulsorily eliminated it should be possible for reclamation and evacuation to go on in an orderly fashion."[50] According to settlement officer J. Griffiths, "bush" Africans choose isolation to escape civic responsibility: "The irksome duties of citizenship are reduced to a minimum."[51] Colonialists argued that drug treatment was impossible because local people did not realize they had sleeping sickness until it was too late and hesitated to go to clinics. As opposed to apologies and suggestions of the aid and compensation owed to Africans, some colonial arguments included calls that sleeping sickness controls make Africans work for their dislocation: "The aim in resettlement has been to alleviate genuine hardship resulting from emigration, but that the settler should not be spoon-fed. After all, everyone appreciates a thing more if he has to work for it."[52] Forced relocation as forced modernization was therefore a moral exercise of colonial power.

A flip side to the argument that tsetse infested areas were desolate with dispersed and transient populations, that land was infested because it was not effectively occupied by Africans, was that relocation was not a burden to transient populations already in motion. The British used evidence of historical and on-going African mobility and environmental desolation to argue forced relocation was not disruptive to local people: "This mobility should be of use when concentration begins. . . . If they move of their own free will so easily, a government-sponsored move won't be such a strain on them."[53] It was important that African mobility was historical and not a result of British colonialism. Colonial texts discussed in chapter 3 linked images of environmental desolation, human immiserisation, random and impermanent settlement patterns, mobility, and African political decentralization and disorganization. Europeans imagined rural Africans as transient, often and easily changing locations. Impressions of desolation and human transience helped to mitigate land alienation and forced labor as morally and legally problematic.

Officers on tour were intrigued by evidence of settlements either recently abandoned, newly relocated, or in the process of being relocated. B. W. Savory, quoted in the preceding paragraph, repeatedly noted in his field journal that since people were used to mobility, forced sleeping sickness concentration would not be a great imposition.[54] In an article in *Tanganyika Notes and Records*, sleeping sickness control officer J. P. Moffett characterized African mobility as "the flitting" and argued, "Such migration means less to an East African native than it does to the European. The native is accustomed to moving house every five or six years . . . . and to wandering in search of a new home. So it is easy to persuade him to move."[55] Furthermore, "clearing land is no problem as the native is used to 'shifting agriculture.'"[56] Colonialists' discussions emphasized that mobility was customary and therefore relocation was "recognized by natives as part of the ordinary."[57]

WORK EXPERIENCES

People experienced clearing work as dangerous and difficult. Camps were uncomfortable. Men were separated from their families and from their own farms and regular occupations. During the Mkalama clearing in Singida in 1940, native dressers treated 4,100 of 31,000 workers (13 percent) for illnesses and injuries.[58] Falling trees injured and occasionally killed workers. Ax and machete injuries were common.[59] Coletha Francisco of Katoro village recalled welcoming men returning from tsetse labor in the 1930s in Geita: "We felt as if they were returning from war. We would dance and yell. It was very dangerous work, like war, and men were hurt or even killed."[60] She did not connect tsetse clearing to issues of health, but noticed similarities between tsetse clearing and other colonial land projects:

> Q.: Why were the British asking them to do this work?
> C.F.: I don't know. It was lands the British wanted cleared of trees.
> Q.: Why did the British want that land cleared?
> C.F.: I don't know. They cut trees to make farms or to build roads. We women weren't told.
> Q.: Were you worried the men would get sick?
> C.F.: We did not think that they would get sick, but that they would be cut or a tree would fall."

Q.: Were you worried they might get bitten by tsetse and get sleeping
sickness?
C.F.: We did not know about sleeping sickness. It wasn't here.[61]

As with resettlement, men resisted tribal-turnouts by temporarily or permanently fleeing and not reporting for work.[62] Particularly when the proposed
clearing site was not in the immediate vicinity, tsetse officials had difficulties
gathering labor and winning the cooperation of chiefs. The Arusha-Usa clearing scheme of 1945 required a work force of 400 laborers at any one time,
but tsetse officials could raise only 125.

Laborers also deserted from labor sites. At the Arusha-Usa clearing, in
March of 1946, 11 workers conscripted for the month had deserted. By the
end of April, this number had increased to 91 desertions. In January 1947, of
246 conscripted workers, the clearing officer reported 131 had deserted or
were "long week-enders." Deserters sometimes took camp supplies with
them—axes, machetes, and blankets.[63] Bazage Kanumi joked, "Tools sometimes were payment for work. The whites had no use for tools without workers."[64] Deserters risked arrest and punishment, but in fact very few deserters
were caught and returned. Punishment was often just a longer stint at bush
clearing.[65]

Workers also resisted on the job. In 1947 labor gangs refused to complete
what a tsetse officer considered to be "an obviously reasonable task."[66] Tsetse
officers complained about worker efficiency. In 1926 the provincial commissioner in Mwanza reported 20 percent worker efficiency and that untrained
and unsupervised labor didn't understand discriminative clearing and were
cutting down too many trees.[67] In 1950 clearing reports noted a 50 percent
efficiency difference between paid and unpaid labor.[68]

The colonial state responded to these expressions of African resistance with
incentives, cajoling, and tightened control. In 1947 Tsetse Department guidelines reduced the maximum number of workers one white officer could effectively supervise to 200.[69] Sleeping sickness officers tried to convince
villagers that clearing labor was their own choice in their own best interests.
Montague reported that he "spoke to them strongly at Arusha . . . pointing
out that no one else could help them if they were unwilling to help themselves."[70] Tsetse officials tried to threaten and entice chiefs into greater cooperation and to present chiefs as supporting the clearing efforts: "Your chief
is wise and sympathetic and will donate 16 cows for meat for the workers."[71]
Colonial officials discussed ideas of docking chiefs' salaries if they failed to
raise labor or limit desertion.[72] Regulations required chiefs to be present at
labor sites to supervise and motivate their workers and to keep lists of delinquent workers.[73] At Kidaru clearing, the district officer directed chiefs to
schedule shifts and turn a copy of the schedule over to him.[74] Tsetse officers
also offered chiefs bonuses of money and cattle for providing labor and su-
pervising successful clearing.[75]

Tsetse barriers potentially benefited some local elite by reclaiming and legally reopening tsetse-infested land and therefore increasing the territory un-

der local authority. They weighed the advantages of cooperating with the state, and therefore having the state extend their territory and reinforce their authority from above, with alienating local constituencies and having their authority undermined from below. Local leaders might have objected if clearing labor was sent too far away to benefit them immediately, or seemed to benefit neighbors to their own relative disadvantage.[76] Such objections sometimes resulted in colonial officials readjusting clearing plans and labor assignments in return for promises of cooperation from chiefs. There were also opportunities for chiefs to accrue wealth. In Mpanda the Native Authority proposed to the Tsetse Department that they be allowed to seize cattle from delinquent taxpayers and men avoiding labor turnouts in order to offer workers the incentive of a beef diet for work rations.[77]

Beginning after World War II, tsetse officers experimented with paid labor. In 1947 in Lake Province, tsetse officers paid labor 12 shillings for 30 days work, with a bonus depending on the amount of work accomplished.[78] The problem with paid work was that if workers came to expect pay, as in Uganda, unpaid communal turnouts would become untenable.[79] Through the 1950s the Tsetse Department continued to rely on tribal-turnouts, but according to a regularized, though informal, labor agreement. Because desertion, for example, tended to peak during wet seasons when men returned home to work on farms, tsetse officials scheduled clearing labor demands around wet-season farming work.[80]

Food, particularly beef, became a standard hidden payment for clearing labor. In 1930 beef rations at Nzega clearing were one cow per 100 workers every 10 days, and a beef ration for clearing workers was standard through the 1950s. In Nzega in 1930, along with beef, the government provided labor with two pounds of cassava flour per worker per day and one-quarter ounce salt per person every 10 days.[81] In 1945, 12,000 men working for 10 days each (120,000 man-days) over a period of several months cleared the Kidaru barrier in Central Province. Local chiefs were instructed to assemble one-half of all taxpayers. Officials told chiefs to have the workers bring their own machetes, hoes, and food staples. Colonial officers provided the workers meat from 200 head of cattle. Each worker was required to work 10 days, and received three pounds of beef, one-and-one-half pounds after the 6th workday and the rest at the end of the 10th day.[82] Colonial reports referred to moments of beef distribution as "beef and beer turnouts" and stated that "evenings of dancing and meat roasting are greatly beneficial to worker morale."[83] Tsetse officers offset the cost of beef payments by allowing Africans to substitute a cow for labor requirements, although this practice favored pastoralists over farmers, and farmers resented it.[84] The Tsetse Department offered forms of workers' compensation. In Northern and Central Provinces, if a man was infected with sleeping sickness, he received money and food for eight weeks of drug treatment. Injured workers received food as compensation, and dependents of workers killed while clearing got two years of money and flour.[85]

MIGRANT LABOR AND TERRITORIAL BORDERS

There was a constant British demand for African labor on public works, plantations, and in colonialist households in Uganda and Tanganyika that was at odds with sleeping sickness resettlement policies limiting mobility and out-migration.[86] Sleeping sickness authorities sought to restrict labor out-migration from sleeping sickness areas to assure the stability of settlements, and also identified migrant labor as dangerous for the spread of the disease, as workers risked exposure to tsetse on their way to and from employment centers.

Government ordinances in Uganda and Tanganyika regulated labor routes and labor sources. During the initial sleeping sickness depopulation in Uganda in 1907, European concessionaires resisted the evacuation of their workers from infected areas. So the colonial state adjusted regulations to allow paid labor into the areas. Concessionaires agreed to house labor outside of fly areas and to pay for the regular sleeping sickness examinations of workers. Workers in sleeping sickness areas also had to wear identification at all times that included the dates and specifics of medical examinations.[87] Similar regulations were made for workers on the railroads and other public works projects. Africans took this dual standard—that only people working for whites were allowed into sleeping sickness areas—as further evidence that sleeping sickness regulations were a British strategy of land alienation.[88]

In 1929 the Uganda Medical and Sanitation Department reported that the West Nile region was an important source of labor, so labor recruitment would not be completely prohibited. The department did close 45 percent of the district to labor migration south. For the remaining 55 percent of the district that was open for labor recruitment, contractors had to get approval from the Medical Department to enter any specific area, had to have recruits medically examined, and had to report all desertions.[89] However, West Nile, Samia, and Kavirondo labor could only work outside sleeping sickness areas.[90] In 1929 the Vithaldas Haridas and Company Estates requested that sleeping sickness officials check to make sure company lands were not in a sleeping sickness area so that the company could legally recruit labor from West Nile and Acholi.[91] In 1932 medical officers examined 770 company workers from the West Nile region for sleeping sickness.[92]

The administration also used sleeping sickness ordinances as a threat to estate owners to keep their lands free of fly brush.[93] Concessionaires resented regulations and interventions into their recruitment and relations with labor, and owners pressured the government to relax controls. In the same year the government adjusted sleeping sickness regulations to allow labor into sleeping sickness areas (1908), they repealed the ordinance that employers had to pay for required worker medical examinations, although medical examinations were still mandatory.[94]

In Tanganyika, sleeping sickness authorities argued that migrant labor was dangerous both because men passed through fly bush on their way to labor centers and because male labor out-migration from sleeping sickness settlements weakened settlers' abilities to establish fly-free communities.[95] Most migrant labor came from remote, impoverished, and tsetse-infested areas. The Sukuma and Nyamwezi were the largest group of migrant labor in the 1920s. Estate workers in Arusha came from the tsetse-infested districts of Kondoa, Singida, and Mkalama.[96] Sleeping sickness authorities tried to regulate labor recruitment, and thus colonial regulations closed much of Nyamwezi to labor recruitment in the early 1930s.[97] The Master and Native Servants Ordinance of 1927 prohibited labor recruitment in all fly areas, emphasizing that infected people had to be kept out of noninfected areas.[98] General Notice 1003 from 1930 prohibited European travelers from taking porters and staff from sleeping sickness areas into "clean areas" and prohibited them from taking staff from fly-free areas into fly areas.[99] In 1936 the medical officer in Musoma prohibited the Majimoto Diamond and Gold Development Company from recruiting in South Mara.[100]

British concerns about regulating migrant labor led to the 1927 division of sleeping sickness areas into "Dangerous" and "Infected but not Dangerous" areas. In Dangerous Areas, people were not allowed in or out. In Infected but not Dangerous Areas, residents were not allowed to work outside the areas, but people could pass through. The Fly Ordinance of 1943 gave government officials power to designate fly areas and prohibit movement to, from, and within these areas; restrict movement to proscribed routes to fixed periods; or outlaw movement completely.[101] Migrant workers also created an illegal market for room and board as they traveled. Regulations in 1927 and 1932 stipulated that medical officers examine people living within four miles of "essential routes," as these people were likely to have regular contact with high-risk travelers.[102]

Gold mining in Geita and Mara relieved some of the tensions in the southern Lake Victoria basin between sleeping sickness officials' interests in local development and the colonial administrations' interests in supplying European businesses with Tanganyikan labor. European prospectors discovered gold in Geita District in the early 1930s, and laborers from Biharamulo, Kahama, and Sukuma migrated to Geita gold mines. The district officer of Mwanza wrote that in 1934 Geita township had been a small village, but by 1936, 100 Europeans and 1,600 African workers lived in the area.[103] In 1952 over 2,000 miners were employed by Uruwira Minerals in Mpanda alone.[104] Immigration, particularly of Sukuma from Mwanza District into districts to the west, became so large-scale in the late-1940s, that colonial officials worried it was uncontrolled and would result in erosion and local instability. In 1941 the state closed Buchosa chiefdom to immigration and in 1949 closed Usambiro, Bukoli, and Buyombe chiefdoms as well.[105]

Sleeping sickness officials recognized that gold mines in Geita and Mara created self-sustaining concentrations and, although they supported the concentration of local people, they saw unregulated male out-migration from sleeping sickness concentrations to mines, sisal plantations, and other European businesses and unregulated settlement as dangerous.[106] They tightened internal policing that regulated out-migration and restricted labor recruitment in remote and small settlements.[107] Officers also sought to work together with mine owners to ensure that compounds were fly free and that workers did not contract sleeping sickness. In 1935 the Kental Gold Mining Areas Company agreed to have some of its white employees trained to give sleeping sickness examinations, to send sleeping sickness cases to treatment centers at the company's expense, and to register all workers at the district headquarters.[108] Mine workers received mandatory medical examinations, and mine owners were legally responsible for clearing fly bush.[109] Throughout mining areas, sleeping sickness regulations allowed only mine workers to live in mine compounds and restricted new prospecting in tsetse-infested areas.[110] On the other hand, sleeping sickness officers were particularly critical of the Overseas Food Corporation's groundnut scheme in Western Province beginning in 1947; the corporation cleared areas with the best soils, but left fly bush.[111]

Mine owners wanted as much labor as possible living near mines and sometimes supported illegal settlements and African businesses that provided services to miners, such as restaurants and hotels.[112] For example, Vincent Olutoch, discussed in the previous chapter, ran businesses for miners in the illegal Nyarugusu settlement near the Geita Gold Mining Company mine. Furthermore, mine owners resented any restrictions on labor. The Labor Department informed the Tsetse Control Department in 1947 not to draw bush clearing labor from Central Province as it was needed in the gold mines and that sisal growers in Northern Province would also be upset if labor was conscripted away from them.[113] In 1954 the mine manager of Uruwira mine in Mpanda accused sleeping sickness officials of harassing mine workers and demanded compensation. A sleeping sickness scout had ordered workers living near the mine to leave because they did not have residence passes from mine or sleeping sickness officials.[114] Nevertheless, sleeping sickness officials tried to accommodate mine owners and minimize illegal migrations by locating settlements near mines or on legal roads leading to mining areas.[115]

The state also used sleeping sickness regulations to capture labor. Railroad construction and maintenance required labor. In numerous sleeping sickness settlements set up along the Tabora-Kigoma, and Tabora-Mwanza railway lines, residents could only legally settle if they worked for the railroad. Since they could not legally live anywhere but in concentrations, sleeping sickness regulations served to force local people to work for the railway.[116]

The colonial concern about migrant labor and sleeping sickness extended to the policing and supervision of territorial borders. In the early twentieth century there were few border controls, and Africans passed easily between the colonial territories of Uganda, Tanganyika, Kenya, and Rwanda-Burundi. Although colonial borders were abstract map projections anticipating spatial reality, colonial administrations were interested in regulating international labor and commerce.[117] The Anglo-German Agreement of 1890 required that all lake vessels traveling between German and British territories be registered.[118] The Germans, in particular, wanted to control labor out-migration from German East Africa to British colonies to assure labor supplies to German plantations and public work projects. Sleeping sickness control, however, beginning in 1908, was an early mechanism for establishing real controls on border traffic.

Regulating fishing, as discussed previously, involved controlling intercolonial fishing and commerce on Lake Victoria. Fishers on Lake Victoria historically moved throughout the lake; Sukuma, Luo, and Kerewe fishers in the nineteenth century traveled to fishing grounds in all parts of the lake and transported fish primarily from the southern parts of the lake to markets on the northern shores.[119] Major market and labor centers at Kisumu, Kampala, and Masese at Jinja expanded in the colonial period and attracted an increasing number of fishers from the lake region. The canoe registration rules in the Ugandan 1908 Sleeping Sickness Ordinances required all fishers fishing in Ugandan waters to register in Uganda and to obey all Ugandan fishing and sleeping sickness regulations. The sleeping sickness control agreement reached between Ugandan and Tanganyika authorities in 1933 reestablished these rules. Fishers from Tanganyika fishing in Ugandan waters or selling fish in Ugandan markets needed letters from their Tanganyika district commissioners to the Ugandan government, then had to register in Tororo, Jinja, Entebbe, or Masaka. They had to abide by Ugandan fisheries and sleeping sickness rules and only fish in certain areas.[120] Ugandan sleeping sickness and fisheries officials did not effectively police fishing on the lake, but they did detain unregistered fishers from Kenya and Tanganyika they found at Ugandan markets.[121]

The flow of male labor between Tanganyika, Uganda, Kenya, and Rwanda-Burundi increased in the colonial period with the introduction of colonial cash-crop markets and work on plantations and public works. Labor from Rwanda-Burundi and the Tanganyika Kagera District went north across the Kagera River to work in Uganda, growing cotton and coffee for Ugandan farmers or to work on European- and Indian-owned plantations, such as the Kakira sugar estates in Busoga. Beginning in the 1930s, Luo men migrated south to work in the Geita and Mara gold mines.

German authorities responded to the 1903 sleeping sickness epidemic in Uganda and Kavirondo by designing control barriers on both the Kagera River border to stop the spread of sleeping sickness from western Uganda into northwest German East Africa and on the Mori and Mara Rivers to control the Kenya–German East Africa border. German authorities were concerned to keep labor healthy by stopping movements of people to and from other infected colonies. From 1905 through 1912, they set up a layered border defense from sleeping sickness, first using forced African labor to clear fly bush along the coast and rivers, then establishing police posts on the Mara

River to intercept people and turn them back. German medical officers tried as well to close the western border with Uganda and with the Belgian Congo and barred people from Bukoba from traveling into Uganda.[122]

After the 1902 Uganda epidemic died out, and after the British took over German East Africa in 1919, the three British administrations of Kenya, Uganda, and Tanganyika were less concerned about the transborder flow of labor and supported labor migrations as both supplying plantation labor demands and supplying men with wage earnings to pay taxes. In the early 1930s, British concerns about foreign labor's spreading sleeping sickness reemerged. Ugandan sleeping sickness authorities were concerned about sleeping sickness caused by a new and virulent type of trypanosome unknown in Uganda, *T. rhodesiense*, which they thought was spreading north from Tanganyika. In 1932 Ugandan medical officers identified *T. rhodesiense* in laborers from western Tanganyika. They asked the Tanganyika colonial administration to close the border by both land and water until effective tsetse surveys and controls could be carried out.

Tanganyika authorities resisted a complete closure of the border. The Biharamulo district officer in 1933 argued that closing the border would "cripple the financial resources of the district." He reported that at least 20 percent of registered taxpayers from Biharamulo migrated to Bukoba and Uganda for wage labor and that when wages fell in 1932, tax revenues in Biharamulo declined 50 percent. Ferry returns showed that in 1932, 23,000 people from Tanganyika and 33,000 from Rwanda-Burundi used the Kyaka ferry to pass over the Kagera River into Uganda.[123] The district officer of Musoma estimated in 1933 that the dried-fish trade to Uganda generated 25,000 shillings annually in the Musoma area alone.[124] Effectively closing travel and commerce between the two colonies would have cost Africans from Tanganyika working in Uganda a great deal of income.

The colonial government in Tanganyika agreed to close all but four Kagera ferries, where they would medically examine all migrant labor moving into Uganda and issue passes. They denied passes to people from Biharamulo and western provinces and to people who had passed through these infested areas on their way to Uganda.[125] British officials in Tanganyika proposed a 14- to 28-day quarantine for laborers before they were allowed to cross the border and a concentration of the particularly infested areas of Uha and Biharamulo to restrict out-migration.[126] Ugandan concerns prompted sleeping sickness officers in Tanganyika to concentrate 55,000 Africans in these areas between 1933 and 1935 and to offer tax exemptions to mitigate out-migration.[127]

Ugandan officials blamed the 1940 Busoga epidemic on foreign laborers and reissued border-control regulations. Three of the first five cases in the epidemic were Banyaruanda workers at the Kakira Sugar Estates, eight miles east of Jinja. Sleeping sickness authorities repatriated the Kavirondo, Tanganyikan, and Banyaruanda workers on the estates and banned all immigration from Belgian territories.[128] Ordinances tightened control of traffic on the four legal ferries over the Kagera River.[129] In 1947, 4,000 workers were crossing to Uganda every month. Medical officers examined all travelers and turned back, on average, 200 per month.[130]

Sleeping sickness controls worked to turn imaginary borders into policed barriers and to try to contain workers inside colonial boundaries. Africans responded to these border controls by avoiding official border crossings, developing black-market trade networks, and not traveling. Trading practices developed in Uganda in response to the registration policies of unregistered fishers selling their catch to buyers with registered canoes, both directly on the water and at unpoliced landings on Ugandan islands. Illegal canoe-ferry service across the Kagera flourished under these regulations. Workers walked off the main ferry access roads to the river shore where local canoe owners transported them across for the standard ferry fee.[131] Labor returning to Tanganyika reported no one in Uganda asked to be shown permits.[132] But controls did decrease the flow of labor into Uganda. Ferry returns of people traveling north on the Kyaka ferry declined from a total of 60,000 in 1932 to under 11,000 in 1939.[133] Colonial officials reported there were cotton labor shortages across the border in 1937 and a severe coffee labor shortage in the Masaka area in 1939.[134] Migrant laborers resented the controls, examinations, and permit requirements, and some sought alternative work inside Tanganyika. There were more men seeking coffee labor around Bukoba in the 1930s, for example, than there were jobs available; whereas with the open border to Uganda, Bukoba growers competed with Ugandan growers for laborers.[135] Border controls seemed to have had some limited success.

SLEEPING SICKNESS CONTROL AND NATURE RESERVES

> The flies have, in effect, been occupying and guarding the country until man shall grow wiser in his use of it.
>
> Charles Swynnerton, 1936[136]

> It should never be forgotten that in the long run the tsetse fly may prove to have been a blessing in disguise. It has saved huge tracts of Africa from devastation.
>
> E. B. Worthington, 1958[137]

From the mid-1930s, in the face of African resistance and the continuing spread of tsetse, sleeping sickness officials began shifting their arguments to emphasize the value of tsetse for nature conservation. In his 1936 book, *The Tsetse Flies of East Africa*, Charles Swynnerton transformed tsetse from a disease-carrying enemy, unifying Africans and Europeans in a just war for eradication, to an ally of nature preservation against African aggression. Swynnerton questioned the basic goals of tsetse control in a section headed "Man's

Right to Destroy the Tsetse." He wrote that tsetse had been saving African lands from African environmental abuse: "The tsetse, it is true, have in the past performed an invaluable duty in saving great areas of country from becoming peopled, exhausted and ruined."[138]

Swynnerton's shift from 1925 to 1936 was dramatic. In 1925 he told the Tsetse Fly Conference at Kaduna that fly control was necessary "to advance the natives in civilization and prosperity."[139] In 1936 he wrote that local people were the primary agents in the misuse of cleared lands: "He is destroying the country he occupies."[140] Tsetse, on the other hand, "are the most potent preservers of the natural flora and fauna." With human settlement instead of tsetse, "most of the plant elements disappear. . . The varied birds of the bush are replaced by a few adaptable species. . . Scrub cattle replace the fat game animals."[141] In Swynnerton's argument, Africans were aggressors against environmental order and were paying the just price for overstocking, lack of erosion control, deforestation, and random burning. Tanzanians created tsetse habitat by burning bush to clear pastures, "but in the act of doing so he forged a weapon that expelled him from large tracts of country when the means of using them had come." Another influential British natural scientist E. B. Worthington echoed this in his book, *Science in the Development of Africa*, as one of the epigrams to this section makes clear. Colonial responsibilities were not aimed at helping local people reclaim land. Until Africans proved themselves capable in proper land use by embracing and absorbing colonial reeducation, which they seemed unable or unwilling to do, forced resettlement and land alienation needed to continue.

This argument paralleled the emerging importance of nature conservation in colonial rhetoric and policy as a mechanism to delegitimize African claims to land and resources in East Africa.[142] In previous chapters, I discussed the influence of conservationists on sleeping sickness research and control and the controversy over game-destruction policies. Nature conservation also helped to resolve administratively the issue of when local people might legally reoccupy sleeping sickness areas. Nature conservation was a powerful colonial discourse that permanently alienated African lands by championing the protection of African wildlife as the primary colonial responsibility. The ideology of conservation declared Africans the enemies of African environments, thus neutralizing concerns that sleeping sickness resettlement and land alienation violated African human rights and victimized the victims. Conservation raised nature in isolation to a universal and transcendent good, while ultimate, and now permanent, authority remained in the hands of natural scientists.

African suspicions that sleeping sickness depopulations were a colonial strategy to alienate land permanently were well founded, as in both Uganda and Tanganyika the colonial state turned fly areas into nature reserves. The overlap in the locations of depopulated sleeping sickness areas and nature reserves in Uganda, Tanganyika, and southern Kenya shows the close relationship that evolved between sleeping sickness control policy and nature

conservation. From the 1930s through the 1950s, the colonial state recate-
gorized fly areas as nature reserves and forest reserves. The areas were already
depopulated, and there were some mechanisms for policing access already in
place. Because fly areas were depopulated, they attracted and supported diverse wildlife populations. Sleeping sickness areas functioned, in practice, as
game reserves, and game reserves helped spread tsetse.[143] As colonial conservation interests sought legally to designate game reserves, fly areas were ready-
made choices, "where protection can be most effective and interference with
legitimate interests of human populations is least likely."[144] Bruce Kinlock, the
chief game ranger in Uganda in the 1950s, then in Tanzania after independence, wrote that tsetse had "long discouraged the often destructive and frequently wasteful use by humans of extensive regions of scenically beautiful,
unspoiled wilderness, the natural home of the great game herds."[145]

The transition from fly areas to nature reserves flowed from the relationship
that developed between game departments and tsetse control departments in
Uganda and Tanganyika. There was a great deal of conflict between these
departments over the issue of game destruction. Bruce Kinlock recalls that in
the 1950s the Game Department viewed the Tsetse Control Department as
"the enemy camp."[146] The legal separation of human settlement areas and
depopulated fly areas resolved this conflict. A Tanganyika government circular
from 1935 read, "Interests of game and human cultivation are mutually ex-
clusive. They need separate reserves . . . where farmers can defend themselves
and their cultivation."[147] Separating authority over settlement areas and fly
areas between the Game Department and Tsetse Control Department was
mutually advantageous to both sides. Beginning in the 1930s in Uganda and
Tanganyika, the Game Department and the Tsetse Control Department had
joint responsibility for depopulated fly areas, and separate game control policies from non–sleeping sickness areas were in effect for these lands.[148] In the
1940s, as tsetse control became less of a primary colonial concern and wildlife
conservation became more primary, it was easy for the state to shift the status
of lands where Game Department officers had authority under the auspices
of tsetse control to formal game reserves.

There is a close correlation between the map of current ecological zones
and protected areas in Uganda and the map of sleeping sickness areas (see
figure 6.4). Game reserve maps from 1935, 1972, and 1992 trace the transition
from sleeping sickness areas to conservation lands in Uganda. The Uganda
National Parks Ordinance of 1952 created the Queen Elizabeth National Park
and the Murchison Falls National Park. Sleeping sickness ordinances had
depopulated both these areas in 1910.[149] From 1925 on, there was controlled
elephant shooting around the Murchison Falls Reserve (then designated the
Bunyoro-Gulu Reserve) to keep elephants in the sleeping sickness reserve and
away from human settlement.[150] The dense strip of nature reserves on
Uganda's western border had also been former sleeping sickness areas.

Game reserves and tsetse areas reinforced one another. At the turn of the
century in Uganda, Commissioner Harry Johnston established game reserves

Figure 6.4
Map of Nature Reserves and Sleeping Sickness Areas, Uganda

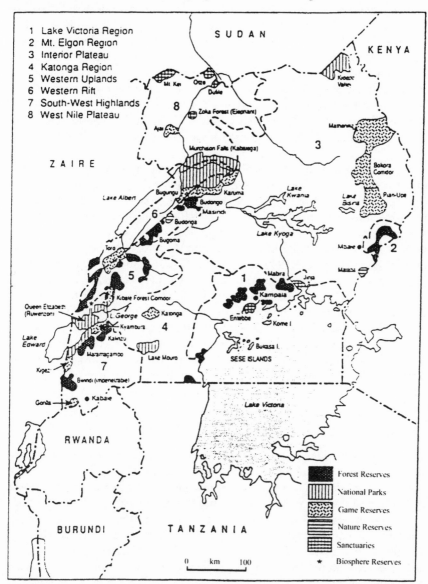

Modified from a map in David D. Gow, *Planning as a Rational Act: Constructing Environmental Policy in Uganda*, Boston University African Studies Center Working Paper in African Studies Number 181 (1994), p. 19.

in western Uganda for the recovery of game from the rinderpest epidemic of the 1890s. Game protection increased the incidence of tsetse. During the sleeping sickness epidemic from 1903 to 1912, the state declared these reserves as parts of larger sleeping sickness areas. As the epidemic subsided, however, the government included areas depopulated according to sleeping sickness regulations as parts of the now-extended game reserves.[151] The colonial state took the opportunity after depopulations to declare forest and game reserves. Sleeping sickness authorities declared Damba Island in Lake Victoria a game reserve in 1926 to conduct tsetse research on hippopotamus and situtunga antelope.[152] The state considered the southern Busoga lakeshore particularly tsetse infested and dangerous and declared it forest reserve in the 1930s.[153]

There was a similar relationship between tsetse control and conservation in Tanganyika. The Masai depopulated the area of the Ngorogoro Crater and Serengeti because of rinderpest and the spread of tsetse. The British turned the areas into game reserves in the late 1920s in the interests of game conservation and tsetse control.[154] Sleeping sickness depopulations played an important role in expanding the Selous Game Reserve, now the largest reserve area in the world. In the 1940s and 1950s, the state added depopulated sleeping sickness areas to the reserve to ensure that people wouldn't move back. The Game Department had the responsibility to ensure "that there was no infiltration back into the vacated areas whether they became reserves or not."[155] In the Lake Victoria basin, the North Kahama, West Shinyanga, and New Shinyanga Game Reserves, founded in the 1940s, were former centers of tsetse control. To the west of the lake, the Rumanyika Orugundu Game Reserve, Biharamulo Game Reserve, and Rubondo Island Game Reserve were all formally depopulated sleeping sickness areas (see figure 6.5).

CONCLUSION

Colonial arguments justifying force and ongoing land alienation as part of sleeping sickness control policies reinforced one another and intersected with other colonial debates about labor. One component of these argument was that in the case of sleeping sickness control, African judgements and actions promoted disease and necessitated interventions in the first place. African opposition to control policies reified Africans as unscientific and reemphasized the necessity of force and continuing land alienation. Sleeping sickness officials at *baraza* offered local people a choice between accepting the arguments of colonial science that they needed to clear brush and relocate or rejecting the scientific argument and thus justify the colonial use of forced brush-clearing labor and forced relocation on primitive, diseased people. The combination of the paternalism of disease control characterized as for Africans' own good, the anthropological redefinition of "forced" and "voluntary" work, and negotiations at points of African resistance structured the practice of

Figure 6.5
Map of Nature Reserves and Sleeping Sickness Areas, Tanzania

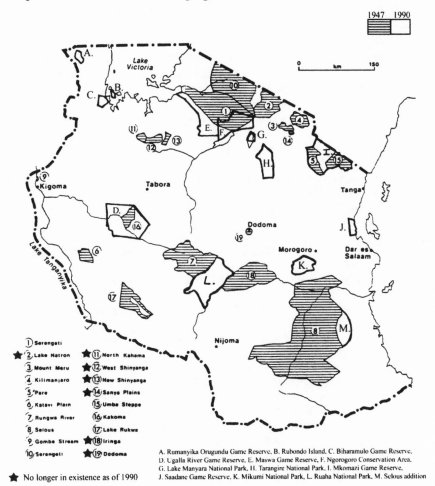

1 Serengeti
★ 2 Lake Natron   ★ 11 North Kahama
3 Mount Meru   ★ 12 West Shinyanga
4 Kilimanjaro   ★ 13 New Shinyanga
5 Pare   ★ 14 Sanya Plains
6 Katavi Plain   15 Umba Steppe
7 Rungwa River   16 Kakoma
8 Selous   17 Lake Rukwa
9 Gombe Stream   ★ 18 Iringa
10 Serengeti   ★ 19 Dodoma

★ No longer in existence as of 1990

A. Rumanyika Orugundu Game Reserve, B. Rubondo Island, C. Biharamulo Game Reserve,
D. Ugalla River Game Reserve, E. Maswa Game Reserve, F. Ngorogoro Conservation Area,
G. Lake Manyara National Park, H. Tarangire National Park, I. Mkomazi Game Reserve,
J. Saadane Game Reserve, K. Mikumi National Park, L. Ruaha National Park, M. Selous addition

tsetse-barrier clearing. Colonial sleeping sickness control through the construction of tsetse barriers continued to be coercive and to influence landscapes and local people's relationship to their environments.

Beginning in the 1930s, as colonial disease controls failed to control the spread of tsetse, a new environmental argument represented tsetse as a blessing in disguise. According to the logic of nature conservation, disease protected nature, and Africans were not victims of tsetse infestation but primitive, irrational threats to environmental order. This new environmental emphasis reinvigorated the sleeping sickness master narrative and the legitimacy of control policies and recast colonialist responsibilities toward Africans. Tsetse control was no longer a noble act done for the good of the primitive but in spite of and in opposition to local people, and colonial officials owed each other no apologies and owed Africans no land. The shift of emphasis is reflected in the geographic overlap between conservation areas and sleeping sickness areas. Sleeping sickness control created both a precedent for and environmental conditions that promoted the legal establishment of nature reserves in Uganda and Tanganyika. Sleeping sickness areas provided the geographical framework for many national parks and nature reserves in East Africa.

NOTES

1. Labor in Sleeping Sickness Concentrations, Western Province, F. Longland, July 30, 1938, TNA, Dar es Salaam, T5/3/215.
2. Interview with Bazage Kanumi, Biharamulo, Tanzania, September 30, 1994.
3. Cooper, 27–29, 43, 212.
4. Ibid., 267.
5. Settlement Officer to District Commissioner Tabora, September 23, 1953, TNA P4/66 Vol. III.
6. S. Napier Bax, Notes on Anti-Tsetse Clearing, #2, January 1932, TNA 29315.
7. Ibid.
8. Tsetse Officer Report, Kidaru Clearing, August, 1945, TNA 24/5 Vol. II.
9. TNA 215/T5/3, 1943.
10. Director of Tsetse Research, April 15, 1946, TNA 24/5/II.
11. East African Tsetse and Trypanosomiasis Research and Reclamation Organization Report from 1949, TNA 37791.
12. John M. Hunter, *Land into Landscape* (London, 1985), 120, 162.
13. Tsetse Research and Reclamation Department Report, 1949, ZA; Labor Commissioner to Chief Secretary, June 2, 1947, TNA 12698.
14. Ford, *African Ecology*, 201–202.
15. Swynnerton, *The Tsetse Flies of East Africa*, 202; S. Napier Bax, "A Practical Policy for Tsetse Reclamation and Field Experiment," *East Africa Agricultural Journal* 9(1944); Tsetse Research and Reclamation Department Reports, 1949–1960, ZA.
16. Director Tsetse Research to District Commissioner Musoma, April 24, 1944, TNA 32535.
17. Clearing Schemes, Agricultural Officer to District Commissioner Shinyanga, April 12, 1948, TNA 32555.
18. John Hall, "Introduction," in *Uganda Development Plan for 1946*, 3.
19. Uganda Tsetse Control Department Annual Report, 1950, ZA.
20. A. G. Robertson, 26.
21. Ibid., 26.
22. Uganda Tsetse Control Department Annual Report, 1956, ZA.
23. A. G. Robertson, 24.
24. Uganda Tsetse Control Department Annual Report, 1950, ZA.
25. Ibid.
26. A. Richards, *The Changing Structure of a Ganda Village* (Nairobi, 1966), 1.

27. Elkan, 19; A. Richards, *Commercial Farming*, 20; R. Mukherjee, *Uganda: An Historical Accident?* (New Jersey, 1985), 191; J. A. Atanda, "The Bakopi in the Kingdom of Buganda," *Uganda Journal* 33, 2(1969); D. H. H. Robertson, "Trypanosomiasis in South-East Uganda," 635.

28. Uganda Tsetse Control Department Annual Report, 1956, 1957, ZA.

29. Uganda Tsetse Control Department Annual Report, 1958–1959, 1959–1960, ZA.

30. Mackenzie, *The Empire of Nature*, 214–215.

31. A. G. Robertson, 25–31.

32. Ibid., 27, 31.

33. Swynnerton quoted in Glasgow, 22.

34. Vicars-Harris, 6.

35. F. A. Montague, Tsetse Report, June/July 1926, TNA 2702, Vol. II.

36. Cooper, 28.

37. G. H. E. Hopkins, "Mankind at War with the Insects," *Uganda Journal* 11, 3(1935).

38. Jackson, 33.

39. S. Napier Bax to Chief Secretary, May 15, 1943, TNA 31598.

40. Swynnerton, "An Experiment," 318–319.

41. Ibid., 322.

42. Charles Swynnerton, "The Tsetse Position Tabora to Mwanza," June 23, 1926, TNA 2702 Vol. II.

43. Ibid., 322.

44. Swynnerton, "Entomological Aspects," 368.

45. Swynnerton, "Nzega," 99.

46. Ibid., 100.

47. Ibid., 101.

48. Swynnerton, "Mwanza," 353.

49. Fairbairn, 21.

50. Maclean, "Economic Development," 45.

51. G. Maclean, *Memorandum on Sleeping Sickness Measures, Tanganyika Territory*, (Dar es Salaam, 1933), 6.

52. Purseglove, 139–152.

53. B. W. Savory, "Safari Diary, Kigoma District, 1934," in Robert Heussler, *British Tanganyika* (Durham, 1971), 94.

54. Ibid., 96, 98, 100.

55. Moffett, "Strategic Retreat," 36.

56. Ibid., 35.

57. F. Longland, "Labour in Sleeping Sickness Concentrations," July 30, 1938, TNA T5/3/215.

58. Agricultural surveyor to Sleeping Sickness Officer Tobora, TNA 24/5 Vol. II.

59. *Bush Clearing Accidents and Fatalities*, Biharamulo, March 14, 1955, TNA 201 T5/2; Tsetse Guard to District Commissioner Mpanza, October 18, 1955, TNA 20321.

60. Interview with Coletha Francisco, Katoro Village, Geita, Tanzania, September 17, 1994.

61. Ibid.

62. District Commissioner to Provincial Commissioner Lake, May 7, 1955, TNA 24/5 Vol. II.

63. Director Tsetse Research to Provincial Commissioner Northern Province, Aug. 5, 1946, TNA 287/5.

64. Interview with Bazage Kanumi, Biharamulo, Tanzania, September 30, 1994.

65. Director Tsetse Research to Provincial Commissioner Northern Province, August 5, 1946, TNA 287/5; Native Authority Order June 14, 1954, Nguruka, TNA P4/66 Vol. III.

66. Assistant Executive Officer to Director Tsetse Survey and Reclamation, August 29, 1947, TNA 34390.

67. Provincial Commissioner Mwanza to Chief Secretary, September 5, 1926, TNA 2702 Vol. II.

68. Tsetse Officer Report, Kidaru Clearing, Aug., 1945, TNA 24/5 Vol. II.

69. Director Tsetse Research to Provincial Commissioner Northern Province, August 5, 1946, TNA 287/5.

70. F. A. Montague, Tsetse Report, June/July 1926, TNA 2702, Vol. II.

71. Provincial Commissioner Lake to Chief Secretary, October 11, 1930, TNA 19094.

72. Director Tsetse Research to Provincial Commissioner Northern Province, August 5, 1946, TNA 287/5.

73. District Commissioner Mpanda to Kabungu Baraza, September 6, 1956; District Commissioner Mpanda to Mpanda baraza, January 14, 1957, TNA P4/66 Vol. III.

74. District Commissioner Mpanda to Mpanda baraza, January 14, 1957, TNA P4/66 Vol. III.

75. F. A. Montague, Tsetse Report, June/July 1926, TNA 2702, Vol. II.

76. District Officer to Provincial Commissioner Dodoma, June 6, 1939, TNA 24/5/II; Sleeping Sickness Officer to Provincial Commissioner Lake, June 2, 1955, P4/61; District Officer to Provincial Commissioner Lake, April 19, 1933, TNA 19094.

77. Native Authority to District Commissioner Mpanda, March 22, 1948, TNA P4/66 Vol. III.

78. Minutes of Northern and Central Province Sleeping Sickness Meeting, March 10, 1947, TNA P4/66 Vol. III.

79. Provincial Tsetse Officer to Provincial Commissioner Lake, August 5, 1954, TNA 30600.

80. Assistant Executive Officer to Director Tsetse Survey and Reclamation, August 29, 1947, TNA 34390.

81. Provincial Commissioner Lake to Chief Secretary, October 11, 1930, TNA 19094.

82. Tsetse Officer Report, Kidaru Clearing, August, 1945, TNA 24/5 Vol. II.

83. District Commissioner to Provincial Commissioner Lake, May 7, 1955, TNA 24/5 Vol. II.

84. Provincial Commissioner Lake to Chief Secretary, October 11, 1930, TNA 19094; District Commissioner to Provincial Commissioner Northern, July 29, 1950, TNA P4/61.

85. Minutes of Northern and Central Province Sleeping Sickness Meeting, March 10, 1947, TNA P4/66 Vol. III.

86. Turshen, 116–117.

87. MO Report, May 1914, UNA; Soff, "A History of Sleeping Sickness," 121.

88. Soff, "A History of Sleeping Sickness," 121.

89. Uganda Medical and Sanitation Annual Report 1929, 57, UNA.

90. Sleeping Sickness Ordinance #93, July 5, 1930, BDA Jinja.

91. Vathaldas Haridas and Co. to Sleeping Sickness Officer Busoga, November 12, 1929, BDA.

92. Medical Officer West Nile Report, October 8, 1932, BDA.

93. "Labor Concerns," District Officer Busoga to Chief Secretary, Kampala, January 29, 1930, BDA.

94. Sleeping Sickness Regulations, April 29, 1908, Secretariat Minute 808, UNA.

95. Sleeping Sickness Report, November 9, 1932, TNA 463.

96. Iliffe, 305.

97. Ibid., 305.

98. Master and Native Servants Ordinance July 18, 1927, TNA 11307.

99. General Notice 1003, 20/9/30, TNA 19097.

100. Medical Officer Musoma to General Manager Majimoto Diamond and Gold Development Co., May 7, 1936, TNA 463.

101. Fly Ordinance #5 of 1943, TNA 29315.

102. Sleeping Sickness Report Mwanza, June-August, 1932, TNA 20909; G. Maclean, Sleeping Sickness Memorandum September 8, 1927, TNA 19357.

103. Assistant District Officer Mwanza to District Officer Mwanza, August 1936, TNA 1022.

104. Mpanda Survey, 1952, TNA P4/66 Vol. IV.

105. District Officer Mwanza to Provincial Commissioner Lake, TNA 1022 Vol. II.

106. District Commissioner to Provincial Commissioner Lake Province, September 17, 1951, TNA P4/6.

107. Chief Secretary's Minute, April 1948, TNA 23892, Vol II.

108. Director of the Department of Medicine and Sanitation to Chief Secretary Dar es Salaam, March 25, 1935, TNA 22866.

109. Director Medical Services to Chief Secretary, July 16, 1948, TNA 23890, Vol. II.

110. District Commissioner to the Compound Manager Uriwira Minerals Ltd., Mpanda, September 28, 1954, TNA 96 P4/6/453; Government Notice #41, February 7, 1942, TNA 26629; Conditions for Prospecting in Closed Areas, March 27, 1946, TNA 23892, Vol. II.

111. Urambo Area OFC Groundnut Scheme Report, June 20, 1952, TNA 40876.

112. Director Medical Services to Chief Secretary, July 16, 1948, TNA 23892, Vol. II.

113. Labor Commissioner Report, April 5, 1947, TNA 35052.

114. District Commissioner to the Compound Manager Uriwira Minerals Ltd., Mpanda, September 28, 1954, TNA 96 P4/6/453.

115. Settlement Report Geita, August 1946, TNA 35052.

116. District Commissioner Mpanda to District Officer Mpanda, March 5, 1952, TNA 28015.

117. Winichakul, "Siam Mapped," 310, quoted in B. Anderson, *Imagined Communities* (New York, 1991), 173–174.

118. 1890 Anglo-German Agreement *Uganda Journal*, 11, 2(1947), 124–125.

119. Kenny, 97–107; V. Ford, "The Trade of Lake Victoria," in R. Steel, ed., *Geographical Essays on British Tropical Lands* (London, 1956).

120. Chief Secretary Entebbe to Chief Secretary Dar es Salaam, February 9, 1933, TNA 215/660.

121. District Officer Musoma to Provincial Commissioner Lake, March 25, 1933, TNA 215/660.

122. Stendel, 434–447; *1904/05 Medizinal Berichte uber die Deutachen Schutzgebiete* (Berlin, 1907), 69; 1908/09, 25–29; 1090/10, 52–56.

123. Acting District Officer Biharamulo, March 9, 1933, TNA 215/660.

124. District Officer Musoma to Provincial Commissioner Lake, March 25, 1933, TNA 215/660.

125. *The Sleeping Sickness Problem in the Western and Lake Provinces, and in Relation to Uganda* Sessional Paper #7 of 1933 (Dar es Salaam, 1933), 2–4.

126. Acting District Officer Biharamulo, March 9, 1933, TNA 215/660.

127. Minutes of the Sleeping Sickness Meeting, July 17, 1935, Tabora, TNA 21712.

128. Mackichan, 52–53.

129. "Tangazo ya Daima," 811/67, August 1, 1940, TNA 330/113.

130. District Commissioner Bukoba to District Commissioner Masaka, November 11, 1947, TNA 215/660.

131. Interview with Alfred Ishaka, Katoro, September 16, 1994.

132. District Commissioner Bukoba to District Commissioner Masaka, November 11, 1947, TNA 215/660.

133. Inspector of Labor Kampala to District Commissioner Bukoba, November 8, 1939, TNA 215/660.

134. District Officer Bukoba to Provincial Commissioner Mwanza, April 13, 1937; Inspector of Labor Kampala to District Commissioner Bukoba, November 8, 1939, TNA 215/660.

135. Acting District Officer Biharamulo, March 9, 1933, TNA 215/660

136. Swynnerton, *The Tsetse Flies of East Africa*, 465.

137. Worthington, *Science in the Development of Africa*, 254.

138. Ibid., 2.

139. "Report of the Tsetse Fly Conference Held in Kaduna, September, 1925," *Reports on Trypanosomiasis in Africa* (Entebbe, 1925), quoted in Beck, *British Medical*, 119.

140. Swynnerton, *The Tsetse Flies of East Africa*, 464.

141. Ibid., 464–465.

142. Neumann.; Mackenzie, *The Empire of Nature*.

143. Pitman, *A Game Warden Takes Stock*, 3.

144. Thomas and Scott, 399.

145. Kinlock, 27, quoted in Mackenzie, *The Empire of Nature*, 256.

146. Kinlock, 241.

147. Government Circular #1, 1935, TNA 19931.

148. Tsetse Game Reserve Policy, 1938, TNA 19931.

149. Pitman, *A Game Warden Among His Charges*, 243.

150. Paterson, 185.

151. Mackenzie, *The Empire of Nature*, 248–249.

152. Thomas and Scott, 399.

153. Watts.

154. Mackenzie, *The Empire of Nature*, 251.

155. Matzke, "Selous Game Reserve," 40; Matzke, "Settlement and Sleeping Sickness Control."

CHAPTER 7

Conclusion

Human sleeping sickness is a disease of environmental frontiers. The disease shifts from an endemic to an epidemic infection in areas of environmental and social disorder where production systems are in disarray. This disarray involves any combination of people moving out of an area and tsetse moving into recently depopulated space, of increased numbers of people moving through tsetse environments as refugees or responding to new systems of labor, or of people moving into tsetse environments and struggling with a disease regime as growing settlement and rural production drive tsetse back.

In *The Role of the Trypanosomiasis in African Ecology*, John Ford presents the effectiveness of laissez-faire patterns of sleeping sickness control in Africa and criticizes colonial attempts at controlled economies of tsetse. Both Ford's vision of the invisible hand and his analysis of colonial control schemes are based on a perceived ecological logic of sleeping sickness: that the disease flares up where there is not enough or not yet enough stable contiguous occupation to keep land cleared of bush and therefore free from tsetse. In these moments, to use the militarized language of colonial disease control, local people on fly frontiers must either attack tsetse or retreat from them.

From within the discourse of colonial sleeping sickness control, while the threat of sleeping sickness always existed on the edges of the expansion and contraction of African settlement, it was not a disease problem where people either effectively occupied land or where there were no people. Colonial sleeping sickness control worked to define and enforce legitimate and illegitimate African settlement, activity, and mobility according to colonial understandings of healthy relationships between humans and their environment. The colonial agenda to organize fly zones as places where health depended on controlled depopulation or occupation created important ideological and functional links between colonial agents and methods not previously connected to disease control and African health. Land surveys, lists of economic activities and household profiles, as well as blood tests were part of a statistical foundation of sleeping sickness control that either denied or forced upon Africans certain social and economic relationships to environments. British colonial states imagined the coercive and territorial power necessary to solve the disjuncture between the methods of modern science and frontier conditions by joining disease control with social and environmental engineering ideologically and in practice.

HUMAN IMPACT

British sleeping sickness control schemes in East Africa often provided the first and most pervasive mechanisms for social and economic intervention into the lives of people living in geographically remote and marginal areas through efforts to control Africans' relationships to environment. The process of enforcing human population relocations, forced bush clearings, and quarantines around sleeping sickness areas entailed British restrictions on Africans' movements and resource use, proscriptions on settlement patterns, and reorganization of labor. The purpose of sleeping sickness controls was to stop the spread of the disease, protect Africans from it, and create safe environments in which African agriculture and livestock production might flourish. However, to ignore the effects and relations engendered and required by British disease control practices in Uganda and Tanganyika in the colonial period would hide the broader significance of their history. In the context of colonial rule, the effects of British sleeping sickness control increased state surveillance, accelerated colonialist interventions into Africans' lives, and restructured African and British relationships to local environments.

The significant shift to planned settlements in the 1930s centered sleeping sickness control within an emerging, inclusive colonial vision of public health. Starting in that decade, British officials began to recognize sleeping sickness settlements as opportunities for them to establish comprehensive control over geographically captive African groups. Officials in Tanganyika and, within a few years, Uganda began to connect the protection of Africans from tsetse in sleeping sickness settlements to a broad array of health measures the British believed necessary for sustainable and progressive communities. British officials planned each sleeping sickness settlement to have distinct and modern moral, medical, political, and economic infrastructures, legal points of entry and exit, education in and policing of agricultural practices, animal husbandry, and erosion control, all as necessary components of tsetse control. British planners argued all these components of a settlement were necessary to achieve overall health—that each reinforced the other—that there could be no tsetse control, for example, without stable occupation, and there could be no stable occupation without erosion control. Various colonial departments were eager to be part of settlement planning and administration, as it strengthened and legitimized their roles by linking them to the promotion of African health. The planned settlement idea failed in practice because of African resistance to surveillance and control and because of a lack of state investment in settlement infrastructures.

African actions in part determined the form and effects of British disease control schemes. Schemes depended on African cooperation on many levels at various points; furthermore they were formulated around a British understanding of African systems of authority and land use. A consistent and persistent African understanding of sleeping sickness control was that the policies were not primarily about sickness or health but primarily served British desires to control land and productivity through increasing personal surveillance of individuals. Thus, many Africans were deeply suspicious that British medical officers did have a secret agenda apart from, and even in diametrical opposition to, the healing mission. For some Africans the (what they perceived as) negative effects of sleeping sickness control—land alienation, forced labor, and hospitalization, for example—simply outweighed British arguments about the benefits of disease control. African stories about trespassing into sleeping sickness areas emphasized Africans' rights to make decisions about health and resource use: "Some of us fell sick and died. But we fished. That is what we did. You belong where you can earn a living."[1] British officials did make serious attempts to enlist Africans' support as they encountered opposition to sleeping sickness control policies and as they came to recognize the need for indigenous cooperation. However, officials failed to dispel these suspicions when they insisted to Africans that unpaid labor and resettlement were simply disease controls.

For example, in Uganda in the early twentieth century, British policy was dependent on the cooperation of Ganda state officials, while Ganda officials were concerned about the British claiming authority over territory and governing the movements and activities of taxpayers in these areas. The British made efforts to explain the scientific logic of control policies to Ganda elite in order to elicit their aid. In 1906 the colonial administration in Uganda published a pamphlet, *Explanatory Address on Sleeping Sickness to the Natives of Uganda Protectorate*, explaining sleeping sickness control in Luganda and English.[2] In turn, Ganda elites relied on the British to recognize and support their authority over land and taxpayers and to pay official salaries. Ganda elite recognized British cultural prejudices and that they stood to gain by presenting themselves to the British as "enlightened" enough to be receptive to scientific methods. Ganda leadership also had a larger political stake in the success of sleeping sickness control, as sleeping sickness areas were primarily at the margins of the kingdom where local people had historically contested Ganda authority. Successful depopulation and control of these lands meant the expansion of Ganda imperial power over its neighbors. In both Uganda and Tanganyika, local leaders also stood to lose authority over lands declared

sleeping sickness areas and over people forced out of these areas. They therefore negotiated in their own interests, navigating between the demands of
British sleeping sickness control officials on the one hand, popular demands
on the other, and whatever health benefits to themselves they might accrue
as part of the equation.

Local people weighed the potential advantages and disadvantages of their
responses to sleeping sickness regulations as well, again with limited regard
for British claims about disease control. Some avoided labor demands and
designated settlements. In general, the constrained abilities of the British to
police African access to sleeping sickness areas, and Africans' unwillingness
to abandon these lands, meant Africans continued to live, travel, and work
illegally in sleeping sickness areas. Local people did redefine their relationship
to British-designated sleeping sickness areas according to the new conditions
of British sleeping sickness control, but African actions did not correspond to
British intentions or commands and required British sleeping sickness officials
to adjust and revise policies continuously.

The ongoing process of African action and British frustrated reaction pro-
pelled further colonial scientific evaluations and renewed environmental interventions. At cleared landings in Uganda in the early century, and later in
Tanganyika and Uganda at sleeping sickness settlements, the British responded to inconsistent African cooperation with a continual recategorization
of lands—that is, frequent redrawing of designated boundaries between
healthy and sleeping sickness areas and alternate opening, closing, relocating,
and reopening of landings and settlements. Resistance and variable, unpre-
dicted African responses to sleeping sickness controls perpetuated a British
belief in the need for continued scientific evaluation and control interventions,
which in turn prompted revaluation and further actions by Africans.

CHANGES TO THE LAND

African resistance to restricted mobility and productivity and British inability to enforce sleeping sickness controls limited the environmental impact
of sleeping sickness control policies. Vegetation in cleared sleeping sickness
barriers grew back often before the particular colonial clearing scheme could
be completed. The cutting of vegetation for sleeping sickness control may
have contributed to erosion problems facing the Lake Victoria basin in Tanzania in the postcolonial period, though a casual observer in the 1990s would
not be capable of visually perceiving between formerly cleared and uncleared
areas and between formerly depopulated and settled areas. A decisive pattern
of environmental impact traceable to this one factor does not emerge; some
sleeping sickness settlements flourished during and after colonial regulations,
and some dissolved. In areas that the British declared closed, farmers, fishers,
and pastoralists continued to use the land according to variable intersections
of political, economic, and cultural forces. However, cycles of changing state

regulations about land use increased African mobility and impermanent land occupation. In legally depopulated sleeping sickness areas, formerly cultivated areas were quickly overgrown, and infrastructure fell into decay. The amount of new investments in labor and resources necessary to resettle these areas increased, and Africans were that much less attracted to the lands.

Aspects of my oral history research in 1993 and 1994 show the connection between the history of sleeping sickness control and ongoing issues of land tenure. Some people were extremely concerned, even at this late date, about the political security of settling and investing in former sleeping sickness areas. Many local people living near the site of the former Busu sleeping sickness camp in southern Busoga, for instance, refused to speak to me or to show me the location of the former camp because of their concerns that the state might contest their claims to land and their concerns that I represented state interests.[3] Local people on Lake Victoria islands and in fishing communities along the mainland coast were also concerned about my questions. In Uganda there is an overlap between the location of former sleeping sickness areas and recently declared forest reserves. Since the 1990s the Ugandan government has been attempting to depopulate forest reserves along the Lake Victoria coast and protect them from human encroachment. Local fishers and farmers are contesting the government's rights to alienate land. Local people use the history of sleeping sickness depopulations as evidence of long-term state ambitions to acquire their land. Government officials use the history of sleeping sickness ordinances to argue that parts of the coast and some islands have never been officially reopened for settlement.

There are ongoing overlaps in Uganda and Tanzania between sleeping sickness areas and wildlife reserves leading to the permanent state alienation of former sleeping sickness areas. In part the overlaps are a result of the environmental effects of sleeping sickness depopulations. Wildlife populations congregated and increased in depopulated areas where there was less human predation or competition with livestock and farmers. Tsetse flourished in these environments with the expansion of bush and wildlife for food. Depopulation, both voluntary and forced, and tsetse infestation reinforced one another in a cyclical manner. Depopulated sleeping sickness areas became overgrown. Transportation and economic infrastructures disappeared. Tsetse spread. This inhibited human reoccupation and investment in clearing and reestablishing infrastructures. As fauna flourished at the expense of human occupation, colonial officials perceived these environments as obvious and convenient locations for nature reserves. Likewise, the increase of wildlife and tsetse in nature reserves meant sleeping sickness was a potential danger for the people living nearby. The British designated lands near nature reserves as sleeping sickness areas and then logically and conveniently expanded nature reserves to include neighboring sleeping sickness areas.

The political and cultural influence of conservationists increased in the colonial period, influencing British sleeping sickness control strategies and propelling a counterargument that tsetse might be "a blessing in disguise" which had been protecting African lands from African mismanagement. In the postcolonial period, conservation continues to be a powerful state tool of environmental intervention. African national governments recognize the revenue potential of Western tourists to national parks, and Western aid institutions, such as the World Bank and USAID, bring political pressure to bear on national governments to conserve natural environments. In location and in some respects in purpose, the regulations and logic of conservation are the descendants of sleeping sickness control. Sleeping sickness control and conservation historically are interconnected methods for the environmental colonization of marginal lands and for the control of marginal people using those lands.

PERCEPTIONS OF ENVIRONMENTS AND DISEASE

The overlap of sleeping sickness areas and nature reserves, the formulation of control policies, the enactment of policies, and Africans' relationships to sleeping sickness control all connect to the politics of environmental perception. The history of British sleeping sickness control in Uganda and Tanganyika is incomplete without the context of how the British and Africans understood relationships between people and environment and what sleeping sickness came to mean in the discourse about African colonialism. In the structure of this work, and in a real way, African and British discourse about environment and sleeping sickness frames social and environmental histories. British perceptions about African environments—the exuberance of Uganda and the desolation of Tanganyika—informed the possibilities of sleeping sickness control. British ideas about African environments and about African relationships to their environments emerged from a mix of British cultural agendas about identity, the meaning of Africa, and the meaning of British colonial occupation in Africa. The mix included British interests in the value of African resources and labor and how Africans acted and interacted with British colonialists to present their relationships to the land.

Images in the scientific and popular colonial literature of sleeping sickness and tsetse were extensive and served as powerful evidence for the British of the lack of civilization and progress in Africa, of the force of nature in Africa, of the necessity of colonial occupation, and the direction that occupation should take. Disease-control interventions served well as examples of Pratt's idea of anti-conquest. Because sleeping sickness control was by definition philanthropic and scientific, colonial texts represented the scientists and officials that carried out controls as neutral actors morally above the debate about colonial violence and exploitation. Observations by British travelers, natural scientists, and colonial officers of Africans' relationships to nature were, again, by definition objective and nonpolitical, but served to legitimize the alienation of vast areas for sleeping sickness control and for the preservation of wildlife.

The rise and professionalization of scientists in the West emerged from this colonial context and from this discursive position. British sleeping sickness control as environmental engineering to separate people from tsetse flies involved not just the empowerment of biomedicine in Africa and the West, but the empowerment of the broad category of natural science and public-health thinking. Images in popular colonial texts—of sleeping sickness, tsetse, disease in African environments, and about the colonial battle with sleeping sickness—and British scientific texts about African disease and environment generated discussions that informed and allowed certain colonial actions. In contrast, African understandings of colonial sleeping sickness control—depopulations, resettlement, drug treatments, and hospitalization—and of British motives informed and guided African actions.

My study of sleeping sickness control in the British colonial system of East Africa demonstrates the need to locate colonial operations within multiple scholarly fields of study: environmental history, the history of public health and colonial science, as well as discourse analysis. Colonial ideas about nature and Africans' relationships to nature intersected with emerging understandings of disease to become central ideological and operational underpinnings to colonial actions. Furthermore, in the recognition that the formulation and enactment of sleeping sickness control involved actions and negotiations between African farmers and fishers, African elite, Western scientists, British colonial administrators, and the public at large, this book insists on understanding imperialism and Western science as interdependent power relationships.

NOTES

1. Interview with Asoman Wandoka, Sigulu Island, Uganda, December 9, 1993.
2. Hodges, *Explanatory Address.*
3. Interview with ten-cell leader, Busu, Uganda, January 9, 1994.

Epilogue: The Current Regime

The postcolonial history of African sleeping sickness control reflects the structures and politics of national and international disease control that are bound to the legacy of colonialism and to the specific environmental challenge sleeping sickness epidemics pose to public-health programs. Reported cases of sleeping sickness in Africa ebbed in the 1960s as human trypanosomiasis surveillance, control, and treatment disappeared from national and international health agendas. From the perspective of health-control institutions, tsetse areas were of relatively marginal political and economic consequence and conditions on tsetse frontiers made disease-control access and testing difficult and expensive.

It is possible that colonial development and control programs had some localized positive impacts on the postcolonial incidence of sleeping sickness, as John Ford acknowledges. However, in most African nations as sleeping sickness control enforcement, surveillance, screening, and treatment declined, the statistical disappearance of human sleeping sickness likely rendered an ongoing disease problem invisible. After the statistical quiet of the 1960s and 1970s medical personnel reported increasing numbers of sleeping sickness infection rates in the 1980s. In the 1990s the World Health Organization (WHO) and Doctors Without Borders both publicized a seemingly drastic increase in the disease and declared sleeping sickness a major health risk in Africa and a disease neglected by medical science.[1] The WHO reported 45,000 cases of sleeping sickness in 1999. Taking into consideration the fact that of the 60 million Africans at risk of sleeping sickness, under one percent of these people have access to testing, the real number of current cases is probably closer to 500,000 annually.[2] Geographically, the WHO identifies epidemics in Angola, Republic of the Congo, Uganda, and the Sudan and high levels of endemicity in the Cameroon, Congo, Ivory Coast, Central African Republic (CAR), Guinea, Mozambique, Tanzania, and Chad. Sleeping sickness continues to be a disease of frontiers where breakdowns in social and environmental order generate movements of populations in tsetse areas. War is a primary cause of many current sleeping sickness epidemics. In remote and war-torn areas of Angola, CAR, and Sudan, medical workers estimate infection rates are between 20 and 50 percent, making sleeping sickness a more effective killer there than HIV/AIDS.[3]

These statistics grid a sleeping sickness control campaign that reflects the structure of global scientific and medical power at the turn of the twenty-first century. The Programme Against African Trypanosomiasis (PAAT) is an alliance of nongovernmental organizations, international organizations, pharmaceutical multinationals, and African nation-states. In 1995 the WHO initiated PAAT in alliance with the Food and Agriculture Organization of the United Nations, the International Atomic Energy Agency, and the Organization of African Unity (OAU). In October 2001 the heads of state of the OAU established the Pan African Trypanosomiasis and Tsetse Eradication Campaign. These new initiatives focus almost exclusively on drug treatment, although the International Atomic Energy Agency runs a program that sterilizes captive tsetse through radiation and then releases them to compete sexually with fertile fly populations. PAAT research and control initiatives are funded and supplied by a combination of private- and public-sector contributions. The Bill and Melinda Gates Foundation established the Gates Consortium for the Treatment of Sleeping Sickness and Leishmaniasis where Gates's computer profits fund research at various computerized international laboratories.[4]

The WHO program relies on the promise of new technologies and drug treatments. The Card Agglutination Trypanosomiasis Test (CATT), developed in the 1970s, makes quick identification of sleeping sickness infection possible. In the 1980s medical practitioners experienced phenomenally positive results with few side effects when treating sleeping sickness patients with a new drug, eflornithine. The pharmaceutical company Merrill Dow (now Aventis) developed the drug in 1980. Because eflornithine lacked applicability and profitability in industrialized markets, Merrill Dow did not advertise or aggressively market the drug. Refusing WHO requests to continue production for sleeping sickness treatment in Africa, the corporation ceased producing eflornithine all together in 1990. Through 2000 no drug company responded to WHO eflornithine proposals.[5]

Doctors Without Borders highlighted eflornithine in its Drugs for Neglected Diseases initiative begun in 1999. In 2000 the WHO realized that Bristol-Myers was producing the drug again for Vaniqa, a woman's hair-removal cream. By early 2001 television and radio media reported the story of eflornithine, Vaniqa, and sleeping sickness. In May 2001 the threat of further bad publicity drove Aventis and other pharmaceuticals to donate large amounts of eflornithine and other drugs to PAAT for sleeping sickness control.[6] Aventis, Bristol-Myers, and Bayer public relations now emphasize sleeping sickness drug donations as evidence of humanitarian corporate policy.

PAAT currently faces a critical lack of human resources for screening and treatment in tsetse areas in Africa. Resources flow to biochemical laboratory research and drug supplies. Yet there are few local medical personnel trained and armed with the new sleeping sickness technologies and drugs. Nor are there strategies for effective disease-control access and implementation in remote and unstable African fly frontiers. PAAT meets certain political and professional needs of drug companies, research scientists, and international agencies but to date PAAT is not generating diagnosis and treatment in Africa. Resources invested in laboratories and research generate a discourse of progress and health without patients. As in colonial Africa, the disjuncture between research and drug development on one hand and disease control in practice on the other hand reflects the distance between the politics of science and local African experiences.

NOTES

1. Doctors Without Borders, "Sleeping Sickness," Special Report, August 1998 (New York, 1998).

2. World Health Organization, *WHO Programme to Eliminate Sleeping Sickness: Building a Global Alliance* (Geneva, 2002); World Health Organization, *Human African Trypanosomisis* (Geneva, 2001).

3. World Health Organization, "African Trypanosomiasis or Sleeping Sickness," Fact Sheet Number 259 (Geneva, 2001).

4. World Health Organization, *WHO Programme to Eliminate Sleeping Sickness: Building a Global Alliance*.

5. Sinia Shah, "An Unprofitable Disease," *The Progressive*, September 2002, 20–23.

6. Ibid.

Abbreviations Used in Notes

BDA: Busoga District Archives
TNA: Tanzania National Archives
UNA: Uganda National Archives
ZA: Zanzibar Archives

Selected Bibliography

ARCHIVES CONSULTED

Busoga District Archives. Jinja, Uganda.
Contemporary Medical Archives Centre. The Wellcome Institute for the History of Medicine. London, United Kingdom.
Oxford University Libraries. Oxford, United Kingdom.
Tanzania National Archives. Dar es Salaam, Tanzania.
Uganda National Archives. Entebbe, Uganda.
Zanzibar National Archives. Zanzibar Town, Zanzibar.

SECONDARY SOURCES

Anderson, D., and Richard H. Grove, eds. *Conservation in Africa: People, Policies and Practices.* New York: Cambridge University Press, 1987.

Anderson, David. "Depression, Dust Bowl, Demography, and Draught: The Colonial State and Soil Conservation in East Africa During the 1930s." *African Affairs* 83 (1984).

Anderson, Warwick. "The Trespass Speaks: White Masculinity and Colonial Breakdown." *American Historical Review 102,* 5 (1997).

Arnold, David, ed. *Imperial Medicine and Indigenous Societies.* Manchester: Manchester University Press, 1988.

Austin, Ralph A. *Northwest Tanzania Under German and British Rule.* New Haven: Yale University Press, 1968.

Bado, Jean-Paul. *Medecine Coloniale et Grandes Endemies en Afrique: Lepre, trypanomiase humaine et onchocercose.* Paris: Editions Karthala, 1996.

Barnley, G. R. "Resettlement in the South Busoga Sleeping Sickness Area." *East Africa Medical Journal* 45, 5 (1968).

Beck, Ann. *A History of the British Medical Administration of East Africa, 1900–1950.* Cambridge: Harvard University Press, 1970.

———. "Medicine and Society in Tanganyika, 1890–1930." *Transactions of the American Philosophical Society* 67, 3 (1977).

Bender, Barbara, ed. *Landscape: Politics and Perspectives.* Oxford: Berg, 1993.

Black, Samuel, and J. Richard Seed. *The African Trypanosomes.* London: Kluwer, 2002.

Boisseau, Tracey. "'They Called Me *Bebe Bwana*': A Critical Cultural Study of an Imperial Feminist." *Signs* 21, 1 (1995).

Bourn, David, et al. *Environmental Change and the Autonomous Control of Tsetse and Trypanosomiasis in Sub-Saharan Africa.* Oxford: Environmental Research Group Oxford, 2001.

Bratlinger, Patrick. *Rule of Darkness: British Literature and Imperialism, 1830–1914.* Ithaca: Cornell University Press, 1988.

Chambers, Robert. *Settlement Schemes in Tropical Africa.* New York, 1969.

Clyde, David F. *History of the Medical Services of Tanganyika.* Dar es Salaam: Government Press, 1962.

Cohen, David William. "Natur und Kampf—Uberfluss und Armut in der Viktoriasee-Region in Afrika von 1880 bis vur Gegenwart." *Sozialwissenschaftliche Informationen fur Unterricht und Studium* 14, 1 (1985).

———. *The Historical Tradition of Busoga.* London: Oxford University Press, 1972.

Comaroff, John. "Medicine and Culture: Some Anthropological Perspectives." *Social Science and Medicine* 12B (1978).

Comaroff, John, and Jean Comaroff. *Ethnography and the Historical Imagination.* Boulder: Westview, 1992.

Coombes, Annie E. *The Reinvention of Africa.* New Haven: Yale University Press, 1994.

Cooper, Frederick. *Decolonization and African Society: The Labor Question in French and British Africa.* Cambridge: Cambridge University Press, 1996.

Cosgrove, Denis, and Stephen Daniels, eds. *The Iconography of Landscape.* New York: Cambridge University Press, 1988.

Cranefield, Paul F. *Science and Empire: East Coast Fever in Rhodesia and the Transvaal.* New York: Cambridge University Press, 1991.

Curtin, Philip D. *The Image of Africa.* Madison: University of Wisconsin Press, 1964.

Dawson, Marc H. "Smallpox in Kenya, 1880–1920." *Social Science and Medicine* 13B, 4 (1979), 245–250.

———. "The 1920's Anti-Yaws Campaigns and Colonial Medical Policy in Kenya." *International Journal of African International Studies* 20, 3 (1987).

Feierman, Steven, and John M. Janzen, eds. *The Social Basis of Health and Healing in Africa.* Berkeley: University of California Press, 1992.

Figlio, Karl. "The Metaphor of Organization: An Historiographical Perspective on the Bio-Sciences of the Early Nineteenth Century." *History of Science* 14 (1976).

Ford, John. "Ideas Which Have Influenced Attempts to Solve the Problem of African Trypanosomiasis." *Social Science and Medicine* 13B, 4 (1979).

———. *The Role of the Trypanosomiasis in African Ecology: A Study of the Tsetse Fly Problem.* Oxford: Clarendon Press, 1971.

Foster, W. D. *The Early History of Scientific Medicine in Uganda.* Nairobi: East African Literature Bureau, 1970.

Gallagher, Nancy. *Medicine and Power in Tunisia, 1780–1900.* New York: Cambridge University Press, 1983.

Garrod, D. J. "The History of the Fishing Industry of Lake Victoria." *East African Agricultural and Forestry Journal* 27 (1961).

Giblin, James. "Trypanosomiasis Control in African History: An Evaded Issue?" *Journal of African History* 31 (1990).

Gilman, Sander. "Black Bodies, White Bodies: Toward an Iconography of Female Sexuality in late Nineteenth Century Art, Medicine, and Literature." *Critical Inquiry* 12 (1985).

Glacken, Clarence. *Traces on the Rhodian Shore: Nature and Culture in Western Thought.* Berkeley: University of California Press, 1973.

Glasgow, J. P. "Shinyanga: A Review of the Work of the Tsetse Research Laboratory." *East African Agricultural and Forestry Journal* 26, 1 (1960).

Glover, P. E. "The Importance of Ecological Studies in the Control of Tsetse Flies." *Bulletin of the World Health Organization* 37 (1967).

Gow, David D. *Planning as a Rational Act: Constructing Environmental Policy in Uganda.* Boston: Boston University African Studies Center Working Paper in African Studies No. 181, 1994.

Grove, Richard H. *Green Imperialism.* New York: Cambridge University Press, 1995.

Guyer, Jane, and Paul Richards. "The Invention of Biodiversity: Social Perspectives on the Management of Biological Variety in Africa." *Africa* 66, 1 (1996).

Harms, Robert. *Games Against Nature.* New York: Cambridge University Press, 1987.

Hartwig, Gerald. "The Bakerebe." *Journal of World History* 14, 2 (1972).

Haynes, Douglas. "Framing Tropical Disease in London: Patrick Manson, *Filaria perstans,* and the Uganda Sleeping Sickness Epidemic, 1891–1902." *Social Science of Medicine* 13, 3(2000).

Headrick, Rita. *Colonialism, Health, and Illness in French Equatorial Africa, 1885–1935.* Atlanta: African Studies Association Press, 1994.

Hide, G., et al. "Epidemiological Relationships of Trypanosoma brucei Stocks from Southeast Uganda: Evidence from Different Population Structures in Animal Infective and Human Infective Isolates." *Parasitology* 109, 1 (1994).

Holmes, C. F. "The Pre-Colonial Sukuma." *Cahiers d'historie Mondiale* 14 (1972).

Hunt, Nancy Rose. *A Colonial Lexicon of Birth Ritual, Medicalization, and Mobility in the Congo.* Durham, 1999.

Iliffe, John. *A Modern History of Tanganyika.* New York: Cambridge University Press, 1979.

Ineichen, Bernad. "The Strange Story of the Bishop's Head: Or How the Sleeping Sickness Came to South Busoga (and Won't Go Away Again)." *Uganda Journal* 31 (1967).

Jahnke, J. *The Tsetse Flies and Livestock Development in East Africa.* Munich, 1976.

Janzen, John, and Steven Feierman, eds. *The Social Basis of Health and Healing in Africa.* Berkeley: University of California Press, 1992.

Jordan, Tony. *Trypanosomiasis Control and African Rural Development.* Harlow: Longman, 1986.

Kenny, M. "Pre-Colonial Trade in Eastern Lake Victoria." *Azania* 14 (1979).

Kinlock, Bruce. *The Shamba Raiders.* London, 1972.

Kjekshus, Helge. *Ecology Control and Economic Development in East African History: The Case of Tanganyika, 1850–1950.* Berkeley: University of California Press, 1977.

Knight, Gregory C. "The Ecology of African Sleeping Sickness." *Annals of the Association of American Geographers* 61 (1971).

Koerner, T., P. de Raadt, and I. Maudlin. "The 1901 Uganda Sleeping Sickness Epidemic Revisited: A Case of Mistaken Identity?" *Parasitology Today* 11, 8 (1995).

Koponen, Jahani. *People and Production in Late Precolonial Tanzania.* Jyvaskyla, Finland: 1988.

Langlands, B. W. *The Sleeping Sickness Epidemic in Uganda, 1900–1920: A Study in Historical Geography.* Kampala: Makerere University Printer, 1967.

Levy, Anita. *Other Women: The Writing of Class, Race, and Gender, 1832–1892.* Princeton: Princeton University Press, 1991.

Lindenbaum, Shirley, and Margaret Lock. eds. *Knowledge, Power, and Practice: The Anthropology of Medicine in Everyday Life.* Berkeley: University of California Press, 1993.

Lyons, Maryinez. *The Colonial Disease: A Social History of Sleeping Sickness in Northern Zaire, 1900–1940.* Cambridge: Cambridge University Press, 1992.

———. "From 'Death Camps' to Cordon Sanitaire: The Development of Sleeping Sickness Policy in the Uele District of the Belgian Congo, 1903–1914." *Journal of African History* 26 (1985).

Mackenzie, John M. *The Empire of Nature: Hunting, Conservation, and British Imperialism.* Manchester: Manchester University Press, 1988.

———, ed. *Imperialism and the Natural World.* Manchester: Manchester University Press, 1990.

Macleod, Roy, and Milton Lewis, eds. *Disease, Medicine, and Empire: Perspectives on Western Medicine and the Experience of European Expansion.* New York: Routledge, 1988.

Maddox, Greg. "Gender and Famine in Central Tanzania, 1916–1961." *African Studies Review* 39, 1 (1996).

Maddox, Greg, James Giblin, and Isaria Kimambo, eds. *Custodians of the Land.* Athens: Ohio University Press, 1996.

Malcolm, D. W. *Sukumaland: An African People and Their Country.* New York: Oxford University Press, 1953.

Mandala, Elias. *Work and Control in a Peasant Economy.* Madison: University of Wisconsin Press, 1990.

Manson-Bahr, P. H. *Patrick Manson: The Founder of Tropical Medicine.* London, 1962.

Marks, Shula. "What Is Colonial about Colonial Medicine? And What Has Happened to Imperialism and Health?" *Social History of Medicine* 10 (1997).

Marks, Shula, and Neil Anderson. "Issues in the Political Economy of Health in Southern Africa." *Journal of Southern African Studies* 13, 2 (1987).

Mascie-Taylor, C. G. N. *The Anthropology of Disease.* New York: Oxford, 1993.

Matzke, Gordon. "The Development of the Selous Game Reserve." *Tanzania Notes and Records* 79 (1976).

———. "A Reassessment of the Expected Development Consequences of Tsetse Control Efforts in Africa." *Social Science and Medicine* 17, 9 (1983).

———. "Settlement and Sleeping Sickness Control—A Dual Threshold Model of Colonial and Traditional Methods in East Africa." *Social Science and Medicine* 13D (1979).

McClintock, Anne. *Imperial Leather: Race, Gender, and Sexuality in the Colonial Contest.* New York: Routledge, 1995.

Miller, Christopher L. *Theories of Africans.* Chicago: Chicago University Press, 1990.

Mitchell, W. J. T., ed. *Landscape and Power.* Chicago: Chicago University Press, 1994.

Moore, Henrietta L., and Megan Vaughan. *Cutting Down Trees: Gender, Nutrition, and Agricultural Change in the Northern Province of Zambia, 1890–1990.* Portsmouth: Heinemann, 1994.

Mulligan, H. W. *The African Trypanosomiasis.* London: George Allen, 1970.

Musambachime, Mwelwa C. "The Social and Economic Effects of Sleeping Sickness in Mweru-Luapula, 1906–1922." *African Economic History* 10 (1981).

Musere, Jonathan. *African Sleeping Sickness: Political Ecology, Colonialism, and Control in Uganda.* Lewiston, NY: Edwin Mellen, 1990.

Nash, T. A. M. *Africa's Bane: The Tsetse Fly.* London: Collins, 1969.

Neumann, Roderick P. *Imposing Wilderness: Struggles over Livelihood and Nature Preservation in Africa.* Berkeley: University of California Press, 1998.

———. "Ways of Seeing Africa: Colonial Recasting of African Society and Landscape in Serengeti National Park." *Ecumene* 2, 2 (1995).

Noyes, J. K. *Colonial Space.* New York: Harwood, 1992.

Packard, Randall M. "The 'Healthy Reserve' and the 'Dressed Native': Discourses on Black Health and the Language of Legitimization in South Africa." *American Ethnologist* 16 (1989).

———. "The Invention of the 'Tropical Worker': Medical Research and the Quest for Central African Labor on the South African Gold Mines." *Journal of African History* 34 (1993).

———. *White Plague, Black Labor: Tuberculosis and the Political Economy of Health and Disease in South Africa.* Berkeley: University of California Press, 1989.

Paterson, James D. "The Ecology and History of Uganda's Budongo Forest." *Forest and Conservation History* 35, 4 (1991).

Penning-Rowsell, Edmound C., and David Lowenthal, eds. *Landscape Meanings and Values.* London: Allen and Unwin, 1986.

Potts, W. H. "The Distribution of Tsetse Fly in Tanganyika Territory." *Bulletin of Entomological Research* 28 (1965).

Potts, W. H., and C. H. N. Jackson. "The Shinyanga Game Destruction Experiment." *Bulletin of Entomological Research* 43 (1952).

Pratt, Mary Louise. *Imperial Eyes: Travel Writing and Transculturation.* New York: Routledge, 1992.

Pyenson, Lewis. *Civilizing Mission: Exact Sciences and French Overseas Expansion, 1830–1940.* Baltimore: Johns Hopkins Press, 1993.

Ranger, Terence, and Paul Slack, eds. *Epidemics and Ideas: Essays on the Historical Perception of Pestilence.* Cambridge: Cambridge University Press, 1992.

Ransford, Oliver. *Bid the Sickness Cease.* London: Murray, 1983.

Ray, Benjamin C. *Myth, Ritual, and Kingship in Buganda.* New York: Oxford University Press, 1991.

Richards, Audrey. *The Changing Structure of a Ganda Village.* Nairobi: East African Publishing House, 1966.

———. *Subsistence to Commercial Farming in Present Day Buganda.* Cambridge: Cambridge University Press, 1973.

Richards, Paul. *African Environment.* London: International Africa Institute, 1975.

Richards, Thomas. *The Imperial Archive: Knowledge and the Fantasy of Empire*. New York: Verso, 1993.

Robertson, A. G. "Tsetse Control In Uganda." *East African Geographical Review* 1 (1963).

Robertson, D. H. H. "Human Trypanosomiasis in South-East Uganda." *Bulletin of the World Health Organization* 28 (1963).

———. "Human Trypanosomiasis South of the Yala River, Central Nyanza, Kenya." *East African Trypanosomiasis Research Organization Annual Report, 1955–1956*. Nairobi: Goverment Printer, 1956.

Sabben-Clare, E. E., D. J. Bradley, and K. Kirkwood, eds. *Health in Tropical Africa During the Colonial Period*. Oxford: Clarendon Press, 1980.

Sack, Robert. *Conceptions of Space in Social Thought*. Minneapolis: University of Minneapolis Press, 1980.

Schneider, W. H. *An Empire for the Masses*. New York: Martin Green, 1979.

Scott, James. *Domination and the Arts of Resistance*. New Haven: Yale University Press, 1990.

———. *Seeing Like a State*. New Haven: Yale University Press, 1998.

Shipton, Parker. "Lineage and Locality as Antithetical Principles in East African Systems of Land Tenure." *Ethnology* 13, 2 (1984).

Sice, A. *La Trypanosomiase humaine en Afrique Intertropicale*. Brussels, 1937.

Sindiga, Isaac. "Sleeping Sickness in Kenya Maasailand." *Social Science and Medicine* 18, 2 (1984).

Soff, Harvey. "A History of Sleeping Sickness in Uganda: Administrative Responses 1900–1970." Ph.D. diss., Syracuse University, 1968.

———. "Sleeping Sickness in the Lake Victoria Region of British East Africa, 1900–1915." *African Historical Studies* 2, 2 (1969).

Stepan, Nancy. *Picturing Tropical Nature*. Ithaca: Cornell University Press, 2001.

Stoddard, D. R., ed. *Geography, Ideology, and Social Concern*. New York: Oxford University Press, 1981.

Summers, Carol. "Intimate Colonialism: The Imperial Production of Reproduction in Uganda, 1907–1925." *Signs* 16, 4 (1991).

Temple, Paul H. "Lolui Fishermen: A Study of Migratory Groups on Lake Victoria." *Proceedings of the East African Academy* 3 (1965).

Torgovnick, Marianna. *Gone Primitive: Savage Intellectuals, Modern Lives*. Chicago: University of Chicago Press, 1991.

Turner, Frederick. *Beyond Geography*. New York: Viking, 1980.

Turshen, Meredeth. *The Political Ecology of Disease in Tanzania*. New Brunswick: Rutgers University Press, 1984.

Twaddle, Michael. *Kakungulu and the Creation of Uganda*. London: James Currey, 1993.

Vaughan, Megan. *Curing Their Ills: Colonial Power and African Illness*. Stanford: Stanford University Press, 1991.

Waller, Richard D. "Tsetse Fly in Western Narok, Kenya." *Journal of African History*, 31 (1990).

Watts, Susan. *The South Busoga Resettlement Scheme*. Syracuse: Syracuse University, 1966.

White, Luise. "'They Could Make Their Victims Dull': Genders and Genres, Fantasies and Cures in Colonial Southern Uganda." *American Historical Review* 100, 5 (1995).

———. "Tsetse Visions: Narratives of Blood and Bugs in Colonial Northern Rhodesia, 1931–9." *Journal of African History* 36 (1995).
Wijers, D. J. B. "The History of Sleeping Sickness in Yimbo Location (Central Nyanza Kenya)." *Tropical and Geographical Medicine* 21 (1969).
Winichakul, Thongchai. "Siam Mapped." Ph.D. thesis, University of Sydney, 1988.
Worboys, Michael. "The Comparative History of Sleeping Sickness in East and Central Africa, 1900–1914." *History of Science* 32 (1994).
Wright, Peter, and Andrew Treacher, eds. *The Problem of Medical Knowledge*. Edinburgh: Edinburgh University Press, 1982.
Young, Allan. "Modes of Production of Medical Knowledge." *Medical Anthropology* 2 (1978).
Young, Crawford. *The Colonial State in Comparative Perspective*. New Haven: Yale University Press, 1994.
Young, Robert J. C. *Colonial Desire: Hybridity in Theory, Culture, and Race*. New York: Routledge, 1995.

PRIMARY SOURCES

Burton, Richard. *The Lake Regions of Central Africa*. London: Longman, 1860.
Buxton, Patrick A. *The Natural History of Tsetse Flies*. London: H.K. Lewis, 1955.
Cameron, Donald. *My Tanganyika Service and Some Nigeria*. London: George Allen, 1939.
Carpenter, G. D. H. *A Naturalist on Lake Victoria, With an Account of Sleeping Sickness and the Tsetse Fly*. London: Adelphi Terrace, 1920.
———. "Progress Report on Investigation into the Bionomics of Glossina Palpalis." *Reports of the Sleeping Sickness Commission of the Royal Society XII* (1912).
———. "Third Report on the Bionomics of Glossina palpalis." *Reports of the Sleeping Sickness Commission of the Royal Society* XVII (1919).
Decle, Lionel. *Three Years in Savage Africa*. London: Methuen, 1898.
Du Chaillu, Paul. *Wildlife Under the Equator*. New York: Harper, 1869.
Duke, H. Lundhurst. "The Sleeping Sickness Reservoir on the Islands of Lake Victoria Nyanza." *Reports of the Sleeping Sickness Commission of the Royal Society* XIII (1913).
Elliot, G. F. Scott. *A Naturalist in Mid-Africa*. London: A.D. Innes, 1896.
Fairbairn, H. "The Agricultural Problems Posed by Sleeping Sickness Settlements." *East African Agricultural Journal* 9, 1 (1943).
Fiske, W. F. *A History of Sleeping Sickness and Reclamation in Uganda*. Entebbe: Government Printer, 1927.
Graham, M. *The Victoria Nyanza and Its Fisheries: A Report on the Fishing Survey of Lake Victoria, 1927–1928*. London, 1929.
Grant, James A. *A Walk Across Africa*. Edinburgh, 1864.
Gray, A. C. H. "Report on the Sleeping Sickness Camps, Uganda, and on the Medical Treatment of Sleeping Sickness Patients at the Segregation Camps, from December, 1906, to January, 1908." *Reports of the Sleeping Sickness Commission of the Royal Society* IX (1908).
Gray, A. C. H., and F. M. G. Tulloch "Continuation Report on Sleeping Sickness in Uganda." *Reports of the Sleeping Sickness Commission of the Royal Society* VIII (1907).

Greig, E. D. W. "Report on Sleeping Sickness in the Nile Valley." *Reports of the Sleeping Sickness Commission of the Royal Society* VI (1906).

Griffiths, J. "The Aba-ha of Tanganyika Territory—Some Aspects of their Tribal Organization and Sleeping Sickness Concentration." *Tanganyika Notes and Records* 2 (1936).

Haggard, H. Rider. *King Solomon's Mines.* 1885. Reprint, New York: Magnum, 1968.

Hailey, Lord. *An African Survey.* London, 1938.

Hall, John. *Uganda Development Plan for 1946.* Entebbe: Government Printer, 1946.

Harrison, H. "The Shinyanga Game Experiment: A Few Early Observations." *Journal of Animal Ecology* 5 (1936).

Hatchell, C. W. "An Early 'Sleeping Sickness Settlement' in South-Western Tanganyika." *Tanganyika Notes and Records* 27 (1949).

Hattersley, C. W. *Uganda by Pen and Camera.* London: Religious Tract Society, 1907.

Hodges, A. D. P. *Explanatory Address on Sleeping Sickness to the Natives of the Uganda Protectorate.* Entebbe: Government Printer, 1906.

————. "Report on Sleeping Sickness in Unyoro and Nile Valley." *Reports of the Sleeping Sickness Commission of the Royal Society* VIII (1906).

————. "Report on Sleeping Sickness in Uganda from January 1st to June 30th, 1906." *Reports of the Sleeping Sickness Commission of the Royal Society* IX (1908).

Hopkins, G. H. E. "Mankind at War with the Insects." *Uganda Journal* 11, 3 (1935).

Hore, E. C. *Tanganyika: Eleven Years in Central Africa.* London: Edward Stanford, 1892.

Jackson, C. H. N. "On Two Advances of Tsetse-Flies in Central Tanganyika." *Proceedings of the Royal Entomological Society of London* 24a (1950).

Johnson, W. B. *Notes upon a Journey through Certain Belgian, French, and British African Dependencies to Observe General Medical Organization and Methods of Trypanosomiasis Control.* Lagos: Government Printer, 1929.

Johnston, Harry. *The Uganda Protectorate.* 2 vols. London: Hutchinson, 1902.

Jones, Herbert G. *Uganda in Transformation.* London: CMS, 1926.

Kearton, Cherry, and James Barnes. *Through Central Africa from East to West.* London: Cassell, 1915.

Kirkland, Caroline. *Some African Highways: A Journey of Two American Women to Uganda and the Transvaal.* Boston: Dana Estes, 1908.

Kollman, Paul. *The Victoria Nyanza.* London: Swann Sonnenschein, 1899.

Lankester, Edwin Ray. *The Kingdom of Man.* London: Constable, 1907.

Lewis, E. Aneurin. "Tsetse-Flies and Development in Kenya Colony, Part I." *East African Agricultural Journal* 7 (1941/42).

————. "Tsetse-Flies and Development in Kenya Colony, Part II." *East African Agricultural Journal* 8 (1941/42).

————. "Tsetse-Flies and Development in Kenya Colony, Part III." *East African Agricultural Journal* 9 (1941/42).

————. "Tsetse-Flies in the Masai Reserve, Kenya Colony." *Bulletin of Entomological Research* 25 (1934).

Livingston, David. "Arsenic as a Remedy for the Tsetse Bite." *British Medical Journal* 1 (1858).

————. *Missionary Travels and Researches in South Africa.* New York: Harper, 1872.

Livingston, David, and Charles Livingston. *Narrative of an Expedition to the Zambezi and Its Tributaries.* New York: Harper, 1866.

Lugard, F. D. *The Rise of Our East African Empire.* London: Blackwood, 1893.

Mackay, A. M. *Mackay of Uganda*. London: Hodder, 1890.

Mackichan, I. W. "Rhodesian Sleeping Sickness in Eastern Uganda." *Transactions of the Royal Society of Medicine and Hygiene* 38, 1 (1944).

Maclean, G. "The Relationship between Economic Development and Rhodesian Sleeping Sickness in Tanganyika Territory." *Annals of Tropical Medicine and Parasitology* 23 (1929).

———. "Sleeping Sickness Measures in Tanganyika Territory." *Kenya and East African Medical Journal* (1930).

Moffett, J. P. *Handbook of Tanganyika*. Dar es Salaam: Government Printer, 1930.

———. "A Strategic Retreat from Tsetse Fly: Uyowa and Bugomba Concentrations, 1934." *Tanganyika Notes and Records* 7 (1939).

Oswald, Felix. *Alone in the Sleeping Sickness Country*. London: K. Paul, Trench, Trubner, 1923.

Paasche, Hermann. *Deutsch-Ostafrika*. Berlin: Schmetschke, 1906.

Pitman, C. R. S. *A Game Warden Among His Charges*. London, 1931.

———. *A Game Warden Takes Stock*. London, 1942.

Portal, Gerald. *The British Mission to Uganda in 1893*. London: Edward Arnold, 1894.

Purseglove, J. W. "Kigezi Resettlement." *Uganda Journal* 14, 2 (1950).

Purvis, J. B. *Through Uganda to Mount Elgon*. London: Adelphi Terrace, 1909.

Reynolds, Reginald. *Cleanliness and Godliness*. New York: Doubleday, 1946.

Roscoe, John. *The Baganda: An Account of Native Customs and Beliefs*. London: Macmillan, 1911.

———. *The Northern Bantu*. Cambridge: Cambridge University Press, 1915.

Schnitzer, Eduard. *Emin Pasha in Central Africa*. London: G. Philip, 1888.

———. *Emin Pasha, His Life and Work*. Westminster: A. Constable, 1898.

Speke, A. G., and E. B. Adams. "Account of a Tour in Northern Unyoro and on the Victoria Nile." *Reports of the Sleeping Sickness Commission of the Royal Society* VIII (1906).

Speke, John. *Journal of the Discovery of the Source of the Nile*. New York: Harper, 1864.

Stanley, Henry. *Through the Dark Continent*. London: Lampson, Low, 1890.

Stendel, Dr. "Der Kampf Gegen die Schlafkrankheit." *Deutsches Kolonialblatt* 22 (1912).

Stuhlmann, Franz. *Mit Emin Pasha in Herz von Afrika*. Berlin: D. Reimer, 1894.

———. "Notizen Uber die Tsetsefliege und die durch sie ubertrangene Surrankrankheit in Deutsch-Ostafrika." *Berichte uber Land-und-Forstwirtschaft* 1 (1902).

Swynnerton, C. F. M. "The Entomological Aspects of an Outbreak of Sleeping Sickness Near Mwanza, Tanganyika Territory." *Bulletin of Entomological Research* 13 (1922).

———. "An Examination of the Tsetse Problem in North Mossurise, Portuguese East Africa." *Bulletin of Entomological Research* 11 (1921),315–385.

———. "An Experiment in Control of Tsetse-Flies at Shinyanga, Tanganyika Territory." *Bulletin of Entomological Research* 15 (1924).

———. *The Tsetse Flies of East Africa*. London: Royal Entomological Society of London, 1936.

———. "The Tsetse Fly Problem in Nzega Sub-District, Tanganyika Territory." *Bulletin of Entomological Research* 16 (1925).

Thomson, Joseph. *To the Central African Lakes and Back*. Boston: Houghton Mifflin, 1881.

Thornhill, J. B. *Adventures in Africa under the British, Belgian and Portuguese Flags.* London: John Murray, 1915.

Tucker, Alfred. *Eighteen Years in Uganda and East Africa.* London: Edward Arnold, 1908.

Vicars-Harris, N. H. "The Occupation of Land Reclaimed from the Tsetse Fly in Tanganyika." *East African Annual* 1934/35.

Von Lettow-Vorbeck, Paul Emil. *My Reminiscences of East Africa.* London: Hurst and Blackett, 1920.

Weule, Karl. *Native Life in East Africa.* London: Pitman, 1909.

Wolf, James B., ed. *Missionary to Tanganyika, 1877–1888: The Writings of Edward Coode Hore, Master Mariner.* London: Frank Cass, 1971.

Wolfel, K. "Viehhaltung in Tabora Bezirk." *Der Pflanzer* 7 (1911).

Worthington, E. B. *A Development Plan for Uganda.* Entebbe: Government Printer, 1946.

———. *Science in Africa.* London: Oxford University Press, 1938.

———. *Science in the Development of Africa.* London: Stephen Austin, 1958.

Index

About the Author

KIRK ARDEN HOPPE is an assistant professor in the History Department, University of Illinois at Chicago.